A Practical Guide to Holistic Health

REVISED EDITION

Swami Rama

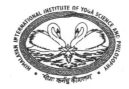

The Himalayan Institute Press
Honesdale, Pennsylvania

The Himalayan Institute Press
RR 1, Box 405
Honesdale, Pennsylvania 18431

© 1980, 1999 Himalayan International Institute
of Yoga Science and Philosophy of the USA

9 8 7 6 5 4 3 2 1

Cover design by Robert Aulicino

The paper used in this publication meets the minimum
requirements of American National Standard for Information
Sciences—Permanence of Paper for Printed Library Materials,
ANSI Z39.48-1984.

Library of Congress Cataloging-in-Publication Data
Rama, Swami
    A practical guide to holistic health / Swami Rama. — Rev. ed.
        p.   cm.
    ISBN 0-89389-174-6 (pbk. : alk. paper)
    1. Health. 2. Holistic medicine. 3. Yoga. I. Title.
RA 776.5.R33   1999
613—dc21   99-35677 CIP

A Practical Guide to Holistic Health

REVISED EDITION

ALSO BY SWAMI RAMA

Living with the Himalayan Masters
Creative Use of Emotion
Freedom from the Bondage of Karma
Science of Breath
The Royal Path: Practical Lessons on Yoga
    (formerly *Lectures on Yoga*)
Choosing a Path
Perennial Psychology of the Bhagavad Gita
Path of Fire and Light 1
Path of Fire and Light 2
Spirituality: Transformation Within & Without
    (formerly *A Call to Humanity*)
The Art of Joyful Living
Meditation and Its Practice
Love and Family Life

Upanishad Translations and Commentaries:
    Book of Wisdom: Ishopanishad
    Life Here and Hereafter: Kathopanishad
    Enlightenment Without God: Mandukya Upanishad
    Wisdom of the Ancient Sages: Mundaka Upanishad

Books of the Sikh Tradition:
    Celestial Song/Gobind Geet
    Japji: Meditation in Sikhism
    Sukhamani Sahib: Fountain of Eternal Joy
    Nitnem: Spiritual Practices of Sikhism

Contents

All suffering that afflicts the mind or the body has ignorance for its cause, and all happiness has its basis in clear, scientific knowledge. —*Charaka*

Foreword

I was completing my fellowship in cancer surgery in 1989 when I heard Swami Rama give a lecture on breathing and meditation practices and their effects on health. Later, as I came to know him both as a teacher and spiritual father, it became obvious to me that all of his teaching was not only practical but also grounded in direct experience.

Swami Rama was one of those rare masters from the lineage of accomplished sages in the East who attained direct knowledge. He taught that the way to health was through a holistic approach, an approach that takes the entire being—body, mind, and spirit—into account. One of his constant themes, both in lectures and in conversation, was that the basis of holistic health lies in our understanding of the purpose of life and knowing how to achieve that purpose. Swamiji often said that the power to make ourselves healthy lies within us all and will manifest if we are prepared to follow a systematic method of achieving it.

In spite of the enormous scientific and technological advances of the past half century, illnesses related to discontent, fear, stress, and unhappiness are reaching epidemic proportions. It is only recently that conventional medical science has begun to look beyond the physical being for the sources of disease. Slowly we are beginning to understand that we cannot hope to achieve radiant health until we learn to attend to the well-being of the mind and spirit, as well as that of the body. In this slender volume, written in 1978 when the concept of holistic health was almost unheard of, Swamiji assures us that we each have the inner potential to be completely healthy and happy here and now. In one of his lectures, in a voice ringing with conviction, he even said, "I assure you that we have the power to convert food into poison and we have the power to convert food into nectar." He knew that when we assume responsibility for our own health and healing we will begin to make the lifestyle choices that will enhance our mental, emotional, and spiritual growth and ensure physical health in the process.

The most important lifestyle choice of all is the choice to have a positive mental outlook. As Swamiji often said, "Attitude is the most important factor in realizing health." As a cancer surgeon I have seen the truth of this borne out again and again. On many occasions I have observed two patients with the same cancer undergo the same successful surgery and treatment, and yet experience entirely different outcomes. Why? Patients who live in constant fear that the disease will recur, those who are depressed and anxious and have a negative attitude toward life, have much more frequent events of recurrence, and consequently a shorter life than those with a positive outlook and a cheerful cast of mind.

I have also seen vivid proof of Swamiji's statement, "It is more important to be free of the fear of death than it is to be free from death. Fear of death is much more painful than death itself." There is no question that the negative side effects of radical surgery and chemotherapy are often more severe in those who are surrounded with negative emotions, especially the constant fear of death. True healing is impossible in an environment charged with negative emotions.

Disease or health? The choice is often ours. This small book, which serves as a guide to the health of the body, mind, and spirit, is invaluable for anyone who is determind to take charge of his or her own well-being. It provides a

simple, systematic approach to diet, exercise, breath awareness, positive use of emotions, relationships, meditation,
and other spiritual practices so that the whole person—
body, mind, and spirit—can achieve radiant health. It is a
source of both inspiration and practical instruction for
those who are truly determined to bring so much awareness, health, purpose, and joy into their daily lives that it
spills over into the world that surrounds them.

Sukamal Saha, M.D.
July 1999

CHAPTER ONE

What Is Holistic Health?

*O*UR MODERN CIVILIZATION claims to be very productive, creative, and resourceful—but a hundred years ago we did not have many of the diseases that exist today. Every day more diseases are being created. For although we are alive, the majority of us experience only the art of existing. Very few of us have really cultivated that technique which is called the art of living. The reason for this is that life today has become very artificial. Man never stops to consider that he may have gone too far by ignoring his natural resources and by depending on artificial means. Living by artificial means gradually decreases natural resistances, and this obsession makes modern man suffer more and more. Man's whole life seems to be kept busy in trying to get rid of self-created suffering. Is there nothing higher for human beings to obtain than freedom from these ailments?

There is no remedy in any system of medicine for such a self-created condition except to be aware of the fact that it is the individual who creates these miseries for himself and that only he can learn how to prevent them. With the bounty of nature outside and the center of consciousness within, we should be living in health and harmony—but having built boundaries, both externally and internally, we have lost direct contact with these forces. All human beings have the inner potential and skill to be completely healthy, but in today's world, because of the social and economic pressures, human beings have forgotten that all things happen deep within before they appear on the physical and mental levels. We must understand our inner skills and resources and use them as much as possible in order to ensure perfect health.

By first paying attention to the physical being, we become aware that all our actions, emotions, and feelings are governed from within by the conscious and unconscious mind. Finally, we realize that the mental aspect of health is more important than the physical, and that the spiritual aspect of health is of greater importance than either of these. When we start paying attention to the various zones of our being and learn to transcend them, the most subtle level of existence comes into consciousness. Ultimately we become aware of the center of consciousness within, that which flows outward in various degrees and grades. This particular level is called spiritual health. Those who understand this are practicing the art of living and being. One who remains constantly aware of this center enjoys all the gifts of life.

The ancients were aware of the fact that human beings suffer on various levels: physical, mental, and spiritual. They did much research, and if modern man would learn how to modify and apply that research, he would not be as unhealthy and insecure as he is today. The Upanishads say that if one possesses both *avidya* (mundane, temporal knowledge) and *vidya* (spiritual knowledge), one can remain happy, successfully cross the mire of delusion, and be liberated. The ancients emphasized the necessity of holistic health—which means to understand the entire human being. This study is as ancient as human life. Only a few texts survive which describe the practical steps for achieving physical, mental, and spiritual health, and these are understood by only a small number of accomplished yogis and scholars. I was taught some of these manuscripts, and I want to pass on this knowledge.

In studying health one learns biological, physiological, psychological, and philosophical concepts—but I want to explain an entirely different concept. I want to discuss holistic health, which includes all of the above, as seen from the yoga viewpoint. I will describe the health practices which have been taught in the Himalayas for centuries, and give a few simple and subtle points which will help in attaining a good and healthy life. In doing this I will examine health on the physical, mental, and spiritual levels.

The yoga approach to health is extremely simple, logical, and practical. It lays stress on the words *yuktahar viharasya*—eating and living as they should be done. By simply studying your own capacity and learning how to regulate your dietary habits, external activities, and thinking process, it is possible to gain control over your life and remain healthy. This does not mean that you must do anything unnatural or impossible; there need not be restrictions; but given the information in these lessons, you can decide what is best for yourself, and implement whatever changes you choose, practicing them according to your own capacity.

The yoga practices described in the ancient manuscripts are not just physical; they are mental and spiritual too, for yoga is the science of self-effort, of self-examination, and of self-awareness. It is a scientific discipline perfected over millennia. The yoga techniques work; they have been proven and validated by many. By sincerely and honestly following these simple rules you will achieve success. As you practice you will begin to see and feel how much you have accomplished through your own daily efforts. You will come to understand the way to attainment.

The ancient manuals to which I am referring explain the science of living and discuss the techniques for extending the life span by means of a system called Ayurvedic medicine. *Ayur* means "age," and *veda* means "science of"—Ayurvedic medicine originated to control the aging process. I have heard people say that they are very intelligent—but what happens to their intelligence after they reach the age of seventy? In our society today people who are over seventy or eighty years old are put into a nursing home. The theory is that they do not communicate well, and since they can no longer care for themselves they are useless and a burden. Modern man loses his intelligence before he gets old—but old people should actually be the wisest and the most capable of teaching, since they have experienced more. In ancient times people did not lose intelligence as they grew old—on the contrary, the more they aged, the wiser they became. This is the difference: we grow old and lose our intelligence; they grew with age and were called wise. They understood more because they knew of the power of living. We have lost this knowledge.

Many modern academicians say people were ignorant in ancient times, but I don't agree with them. The ancients knew much about life. What is more, their science was very sophisticated. Surgical operations, for instance, were being performed successfully by Indian physicians hundreds of years ago, and the Chinese knew about the principles of vaccination centuries before Edward Jenner's "revolutionary" discovery.

Yet despite these skills, the ancients did not disregard the importance of prevention. The major emphasis of the ancient texts is on a holistic approach. Diet and proper elimination were stressed. Correct breathing and self-control were taught, and the influence of climate was carefully considered. Their therapies were tailored to fit the requirements and the constitution of the individual. Because ancient medicine emphasized prevention rather than "druggation," modern science is only now beginning to verify their findings.

Unfortunately, most modern researchers still believe in replacement, not in prevention. They would rather spend billions of dollars looking for the cure for cancer, or a way to successfully replace a diseased heart with that of a monkey, than understand the laws of health and wellness. They do not realize that preventive medicine is the best, the easiest, and the most rewarding approach. Getting sick and then getting rid of sickness is a painful experience as well as a waste of time and energy. One should learn to look after the body so that it does not become a source of constant pain and misery. One should cultivate and practice those skills which ensure health, rather than fall victim to those which perpetuate disease.

There are two ways of doing this—one is external and the other is internal. Most of us look after our health by depending on the external sources, but physical health means much more than merely developing huge muscles, or eating the proper diet, or even taking super-fortified vitamin-and-mineral supplements. For if we learn to develop only our muscles and do not realize our mental capacities, then for lack of this mental willpower and inner strength we suffer and always remain cowardly and insecure. Pain, fear, and suffering will continue to exist, so it is important for us to be aware of the internal environment and not to be solely dependent on the external one, for it is inner contentment and mental satisfaction which are the real keys to health.

The time has come for man to realize that he is not a body alone: he is also a breathing being, and a thinking being—a unique individual made up of complex emotions, appetites, and desires. So even if one were to spend years studying nutrition and physiology, or even go through medical school, the knowledge one would gain would be neither completely satisfying nor completely useful in helping to maintain perfect health. This is because that which is related to the body, that which is material, is not all there is. The body is merely a covering outside the mind, and the mind is a covering outside the center of consciousness within. It is very important to be aware that the body is a tool and not the entire self. Although the body is the most gross tool, it is the instrument used in day-to-day life, and through it one learns many things. So it is still very important and necessary, and must be properly taken care of.

With the body's help man can fly to the moon—but he cannot fathom the deepest levels of his own consciousness. As long as his consciousness remains arrested in body-awareness, man will not achieve any other level of consciousness. As long as he identifies with his body only, it will create many problems and obstacles for him. It is only after the body is transformed to a useful tool that it can be used as a means for right expression and for communicating with others. Often when the body is sick we begin to pay so much attention to it that we cannot communicate with others as we should. For when our body experiences pain, all we can do is focus on the pain. Instead of gaining knowledge, we have pain. We cannot share the pain with anyone else, not even those with whom we share our joy. No matter how much others love us, they cannot share our pain; they can only console us by diverting our mind.

Life means relationships, and without communication,

relationships and life will both crumble. Without a healthy mind it is not possible for a good body to become a good tool for communication. Even modern athletes are becoming aware that without a sound mind it is difficult to have a good body. Interaction with others needs a healthy body and a sound mind. An unhealthy body keeps the mental faculties busy on the physical level only, and one cannot think of anything else but one's body. Pain implies selfishness: it is impossible to care about another when one is continuously in pain. Every human being has something to offer to others—and if we are not capable of offering our services to others because of pain, then we are unhealthy. To eliminate the pain we must find another dimension of life, higher than the body.

When we start to analyze ourselves, start to understand ourselves, we know that we are not the body alone. We have lived with the body so much, and have been told so often that our body is who we are, that we constantly identify with it. This belief is so strong that no matter how much we read or study, no matter how much someone teaches us differently, our entire consciousness comes back to the body alone.

Actually the body is nothing more than an airport where the plane called the inner being lands. Stop reading for a moment while you try to get out of your chair. Watch carefully. You will soon realize that it is not your body which does the standing, but it is something else within that orders the mass of flesh and bones to stand. The body is merely an instrument which obeys orders.

When we examine ourselves carefully we find that there is a center within that has the power to make us stand firmly, to sit quietly, to move or to wait. This center has the potential to be our greatest ally or our worst enemy; it is the source of health or dis-ease.

Attitude is the most important factor in realizing health. Many people actually want to be unhealthy, sad, and miserable. They develop that tendency more and more until they create that personality for themselves. Later on they become helpless and do not want to accept the fact that they themselves are responsible for their ill health. It is important for people to become aware of the fact that staying healthy is not merely a matter of good diet, of taking vitamins, and of doing proper physical exercise. More crucial than any of these factors is keeping a healthy state of mind.

Good mental health cannot be disturbed, no matter what happens. Many people today say that they spend so much time eating, sleeping, talking to others, and carrying out other duties that it is not possible for them to attain the goal of human life in this lifetime. So they want to know about previous lives in order to understand their link with the past. It is a natural tendency of human beings to brood on past experiences. It is also their nature to imagine what the future might hold for them. But when they spend so much time thinking about the past or worrying about the future, they never learn how to be here and now. They cannot understand it; they cannot realize it; and no one can teach them how to be here and now. The moment they think of now, it is no longer there: one cannot think of now and live in the now at the same time.

But once we understand what "now" means, we come out of the past and future and learn to live in the present. Those who learn to live in the moment and have a purpose do not know what sadness is, nor do they sway with the moods or phases of life.

There are three categories of people traveling through the procession of life: time-oriented, goal-oriented, and purpose-oriented. Time-oriented people move in the world without understanding why they are moving. They do not have any true vision of the future. They spend their lives fantasizing some idyllic future or analyzing triumphs or defeats from the past. They lack a sense of discipline and purpose. Because they are continually living in their projections of the way things might have been, or could be, they fail to appreciate things the way they are, and are thus forever dissatisfied. For such people, staying healthy and finding success is difficult.

The second category of people is those who are goal-oriented. They can physically and mentally discipline themselves to a certain extent, and they can conduct their duties according to circumstances, but their vision remains limited. Their goals are confined to worldly attainments such as "I will have a house, a wife, a car, a job, and many other comforts." For lack of a higher purpose their lives remain oriented toward material goals. They think that these things will satisfy them and fulfill the purpose of life—but after attaining them, they feel lost because they do not know why they had sought them in the first place.

The third category of people is composed of those few individuals who are purpose-oriented: whatever they think, speak, and do is in accordance with their purpose in life. They regulate their habits and know that physical and mental health are not two different things, but are inseparable units which are essential for maintaining holistic health. For them maintaining good physical and mental health is like preserving two fine instruments which can be used to carry out the purpose of life. What label one attaches to this purpose—happiness, perfection, health, a state of tranquility, nirvana, samadhi, Godhead—is immaterial. The people of this last category are rare, but they are healthy in all respects.

Thus it is clear that the basis of holistic health lies in

understanding the purpose of life and learning how to achieve that purpose. There are many questions human beings want to answer. However, it is only when they are sick or when they don't have all the normal amenities of life or when they are befallen by a personal tragedy that they begin asking "Why am I here? What is the purpose of my life? From where have I come? Where will I go?" These are not cultural questions; they are not social or economic questions, either. These are inborn questions common to every human being, and they arise when one starts examining life. Everyone has to face these questions sooner or later. Without answers to these questions, mere physical health or mental soundness will not fulfill the purpose of life. An emptiness, a void, and a feeling of dissatisfaction within will still remain.

For instance, after attempting many experiments along the path of happiness, couples frequently do not know why they are still unhappy. Although they live together, love each other, are sincere and honest, and do their duties, they are not fully satisfied. They do not know why they are unhappy, because they still do not know the purpose of their lives. It is very important to realize the source of their unhappiness so that their unconscious minds do not create problems and keep them from being free.

For if we know where we have come from and why we have come, and if we have no fear of death, then we will enjoy life, even on the sensory level. Commonly people cannot really enjoy their pleasures, because they are more concerned with their fears. They worry "What will happen if this thing is snatched from me? What will happen if one of us dies? What will happen if something suddenly occurs?" Fear is our greatest enemy, and if allowed to develop excessively, it even threatens our sense of self-preservation. To succumb to fear is like committing suicide. But with human beings there is always fear, always something that does not allow us to fully enjoy life's privileges. Only when we can attain a state which is free from fear can we enjoy all things within and without.

I am not talking about emotional or ignorant fearlessness. (For instance, I once saw a bull rush in anger to attack an oncoming train. He killed himself, of course.) I am talking about that fearlessness which can be attained by understanding life as much as possible through mental concepts and behavior. Human beings are perfectly equipped with all the necessary resources to attain this state of fearlessness—and happiness, wisdom, and enlightenment can only be achieved from that state. Otherwise, happiness is only a word that you know how to spell; you cannot understand what happiness really is until you attain freedom from all anxieties.

To achieve this understanding you must have a practical philosophy of life. This begins to evolve the moment you realize that it has been missing. Buddha developed a very practical approach to life. He said there are four noble truths; if you become aware of them you will be able to understand the whole philosophy of human life. Buddha says first that you have to accept that there is misery in life. Don't ignore it; instead analyze and understand it. Second, he says that misery has a cause. Third, he says that there is a way of eliminating the cause. And fourth, he claims that there is a state which is free from all miseries. But as long as the human mind is going through pain and misery, it can never realize the truth. So Buddha says that if you learn to face life's miseries and become a witness rather than a victim, then you will begin to enjoy life.

There is nothing higher than life itself. The best enjoyment in the world is in life, not in the objects of the world. You worry a great deal about the world and about others, but do not have any awareness of what is happening within. You should be aware that there is something called misery accompanied by pain and that you are afraid of this misery. Refusal to accept that which opposes or upsets you leads to developing defense mechanisms. But by becoming an observer of life, acceptance of its misery becomes possible. The problem starts when you do not accept pain, misery, problems, conflicts, or anything uncomfortable. You should learn to accept these things and then deal with them.

All the ancient scriptures and great men of the world teach how to attain that spirit of mind which is balanced and tranquil. Why should it not be possible to attain this level of understanding? If someone has done something in the past, someone can do it today; and if someone can do it today, then everyone can. But you need to systematize this knowledge. You must first understand and then apply those techniques which will help you attain this state of perfect health.

Unfortunately our present-day models of health and therapeutics, such as modern psychotherapy, lack certain vital principles of holism. The holistic approach should be educational, teaching you methods to improve your own physical and emotional state. Holistic therapy should be individualized, equipping you with a comprehensive program which will allow you to grow and expand your awareness, and provide you with the strength needed to prevent you from slipping back into the grooves of your old habits.

These skills must be self-learned and self-practiced. You should not have to depend on the therapist for motivation; it should come from within. As you perfect the methods of self-examination, self-analysis, self-control, and self-awareness, you become more independent and better able to handle the day-to-day problems of life. Most importantly, you also learn how to transform your inner personality, and this will lead to a state of freedom from all pain and misery.

How do you go about attaining this state of health? The first step is to learn to accept that which makes you unhappy, for only then can you build a positive attitude. Learning to accept those aspects of the personality which cause unhappiness will lead to an understanding of the sources of misery. And it is only after this understanding and acceptance that you can begin to consciously make positive changes and reconstruct habits.

The next step in freeing yourself from pain and misery and attaining a tranquil mind is to never make rigid rules for yourself without examining your physical and mental capacity. For example, you may make it a rule that you are not going to eat at night. That night you wake up with an unrelenting craving to eat. Although you have made a promise to yourself, you find that urge overpowering, and finally give in: you go to the refrigerator and start eating. You feel guilty about being weak-willed, and this further increases your appetite and your food intake. You wake up the next morning feeling sick and disgusted with yourself. You think you will never have the strength to resist your temptations, and therefore you stop trying.

Rather than accept guilt and defeat, you should learn not to have unrealistic expectations of yourself or of others. If you make your program realistic, then you will be encouraged. If you set simple, realistic goals, then you will succeed. Your willpower will not be dissipated, and you can watch your progress every day. Dissipation of willpower is disastrous. The more the mind is dissipated, the more the willpower is weakened. A one-pointed mind creates a dynamic will. Without understanding your own capacity, you start expecting too much from others and from yourself. You should start by developing the ability to examine yourself, for only then can you learn to be aware of your own capacity.

Next, you should have your own thoughts, independent of culture and religion, and from these you should develop a philosophy of life which is simple and direct. You should be flexible and adaptable, able to meet the demands of the moment. You should avoid being too rigid. Rigidity cuts off the spontaneous flow of memory, and then that which you really know cannot come forward. Actually, it is not difficult to know again that which is already known. If you want to know, just know: if you don't resist, then you will know it. It is the barriers and resistances which keep you from realizing that which you already know.

Human beings do not actually need any enlightenment. Everyone says that they want to be enlightened, but wise people say "No, you claim that you want enlightenment, but your thoughts and actions lead you toward hindrances. Remove those attachments and you are already enlightened." Between you and reality there stands a wall, and when you start examining that wall you find that one of the stones of its foundation is the fear which is deep-rooted within. You should learn to be free of it, but for that learning you must not make any rigid rules for yourself.

There are countless laws which govern this human life, and many of them as yet are unknown. For instance, ask any physicist why electrons move toward protons and why protons go toward the center. The physicist cannot reply; he doesn't know. Yet as you begin to explore inwardly, uncovering what is already within, you will begin to see, experience, and understand the fundamental laws of nature. By delving further into yourself, even the subtler laws will come into awareness. Then nothing will be impossible. The great sages who achieved special powers simply understood the more subtle laws of nature. Their abilities are not gifts; human life is the only gift. What the sages did was cultivate knowledge; then they gained control through a grasp of the subtle laws.

Each person should fix a plan for himself or herself. Many people don't make any plans, and if they don't, they can accomplish nothing; they cannot develop their will-power. You should have a program for life and should work for that. That is how to build. To work endlessly for nothing is not growth—but if you work for something and have a program to think of for tomorrow, then life becomes a beautiful poem.

There are many abilities at your disposal which can be consciously cultivated to achieve freedom from all pains, miseries, diseases, and disorder. These are described in the ancient scriptures. But the idea of holistic health should not be buried in books: it should be brought into practical use in order to build a healthy society. This is possible and can be achieved by applying these truths in a systematic way. The process begins by gaining control over the laws governing our bodies. This is the first level of this knowledge.

CHAPTER TWO

Cleansing

*T*HE ANCIENT YOGA MANUSCRIPTS describe two sets of mechanisms in the human body: one for cleansing the body, the other for nourishing it. They work together in harmony, balancing each other. In explaining ways to make the body healthy, the yoga manuals first discuss those systems which are busy in cleansing the body: the lungs, pores, kidneys, and bowels. You should watch and see that the lungs expand rhythmically, that the pores are functioning properly, that the kidneys are operating normally, and that the bowels move regularly. You should try to understand your natural cleansing systems and learn to control and assist them—because if the cleansing systems are not functioning properly, the nourishing systems cannot do their work; the body will begin to break down. For instance, you cannot inhale unless you have first exhaled. If you have not moved your bowels, if you have not expelled that waste, then you cannot enjoy eating your meal. Resistance and irregularity create disorders and disease in the body, and if the body is in discomfort and disease, the mind also remains under stress and the nervous system in tension.

You don't have to be highly educated to understand the nature of the body's systems. For instance, if you have to move your bowels, it is obvious that delaying is not a good thing. And yet I have seen very educated people, even doctors, who obstruct this cleansing process. This is not healthy. To build a healthy body you have to cultivate certain habits which will cooperate with the natural processes of the body. You should not be lazy. You should learn to regulate your habits and learn to be consistent, mindful, and moderate.

There are a few very simple exercises designed to maintain the strength of the four excretory systems of the body. Although all exercises mentioned in the yoga manuals are important, the most important ones described are those that have to do with regulating the motion of the lungs. It is important to understand why you should practice these various breathing exercises, for breathing is more important than eating. There are yoga manuals which are totally devoted to the science of the breath, for proper regulation of the breath is the basis of good health. The breath is the bridge between body and mind. It is the subtle thermometer which registers the conditions of both body and mind. The breath is the source of life. You can live weeks without food, days without water, but only minutes without breathing. Proper breathing is the key to good health.

Modern scientists are only now beginning to understand the relationship of breath control with body physiology. It has been demonstrated that by practicing simple breathing exercises you can control the heart rate, skin temperature, digestive organs, and other functions which were until recently thought to be beyond the control of the conscious mind. The yogis, however, have known and practiced these skills for thousands of years.

The breath is a vehicle for the energy called prana, and

inhalation and exhalation constantly function like two caretakers in the City of Life. The exhalation expels the used-up gases, and the inhalation supplies the vital energy—prana—from the atmosphere. If you can regulate the motion of the lungs you can protect yourself from many diseases and maintain an even emotional balance. Alternate nostril breathing has been found very useful in dealing with nervous disorders, and deep, even breathing can help in relaxing tension. Again, modern research has now verified this, and people have been cured of hypertension, tension headaches, and anxiety states simply by learning to practice diaphragmatic breathing and relaxation. Therefore, just as you take care of your diet, so should you take care of your breathing habits.

You should be aware of inhalation and exhalation and make sure that they are regulated properly, for this will clean the lungs. The ancients mention varieties of breathing techniques they experimented with and found useful in producing these effects. These include *nadi shodhanam, kapalabhati, bhastrika*, and many others. Anyone can practice the simpler breath-awareness exercises, but the more advanced techniques, those using breath retention, should be practiced under the strict guidance of a competent teacher.

You should start learning to regulate the breath by practicing diaphragmatic breathing. If you learn to use this method you will be able to control the motion of the lungs, which work in the body like the flywheel of a machine. The diaphragm is a dome-shaped muscle located under the lungs. You inhale by contracting or pulling down the diaphragm. This downward pressure forces the abdomen outward and sucks air into the lungs. Relaxing the diaphragm allows it to float up to its original position. When this happens, the air is expelled. By properly regulating the movement of the diaphragm you can induce a profound physical relaxation and a deep feeling of calmness; you can cool down an overcharged body, and turn off the internal stress response.

The habit of breathing in this way can be formed by paying attention to the diaphragmatic movement for a few days. You can easily observe this movement if you lie down on your back and place one hand on the chest and the other on the abdomen. As you breathe, try to imagine that you are inhaling air into the abdomen and pelvic area. If this is done properly the hand on the chest should not move, while the hand on the abdomen should rise with the inhalation and fall with the exhalation. This can also be practiced standing: keeping the head, neck, and trunk straight, place a hand on your abdomen and watch the movement of the diaphragm. Gently push in and exhale; then let the abdomen come out and inhale. Fill the lungs, but don't overdo it.

If you start using the diaphragm to breathe, it will become a habit in ten days' time. Practice every day for a few minutes in the morning and the evening; it will help you to perfect a habit that will become a meaningful part of your life. Breathing diaphragmatically may be one of the most important of all conscious acts, as it is certain to produce a sense of tranquility and reduce stress and tension; it could add years to your life.

There are four basic things to watch for in learning to breathe properly. First, you should learn to fully fill the lungs with each breath. Learn to breathe deeply; it is very simple if you are aware of what you are doing. In breathing deeply you can use your full lung capacity, and slowly you will find that this capacity is increasing.

Secondly, as you practice breathing you should be sure that you are not creating a long pause between the inhalation and the exhalation. This is very important: you can form bad habits if you are not cautious and aware. For instance, a pause that takes any longer than the blink of an eye is a sign of a poor breathing system. At the Himalayan Institute research has been done to chart breathing patterns. It has been discovered that anyone who creates a long pause after expiration either already has certain symptoms of heart disease or is predisposed to the future development of coronary disease.

The third thing to observe in the breath is the regular flow of the inhalation and exhalation. The breath should be smooth; there should be no jerks in the breathing. If someone receives a mental or emotional shock, it will be recorded in the breath as a jerk. Thus emotional reaction can disturb the motion of the lungs and the pumping station of the heart. That, in turn, will disturb the vagus nerve and the rest of the involuntary nervous system. When the breath flows smoothly, relaxation occurs; when it is irregular, the body cannot rest. By watching a baby deep in sleep and observing the rhythmic motion of its abdomen you can see how to perform proper breathing.

Lastly, you should watch for noisy breathing, which is a sign of obstruction in the nostrils. The breath should be silent, without turbulence. If done correctly you will notice a sensation of coolness at the tips of the nostrils upon inhalation, and a feeling of warmth on exhalation. If there is an obstruction in the nostrils, and it is allowed to continue, then you will start inhaling through the mouth, which is not healthy as a normal practice.

Furthermore, there are some things that anatomy does not teach us. One of these is that breathing through the left nostril is different from breathing through the right nostril. This is due to the tiny nerve endings at the base of the nose. These nerve endings connect directly to the brain and are stimulated by smell and also by the flow of the air as it passes by. Thus air flowing through the left nostril will cause nervous impulses to be sent to one part of the brain, signaling restfulness and calmness, while when right-nostril breathing predominates the body is prepared for more active processes, such as digestion. It has been scientifically accepted that if one of your nostrils remains continually blocked you will frequently experience pain and headaches. What is more, when the discharge from both nostrils has been examined it has been discovered that they have different electrical potentials—one being positive and the other being negative.

The nostrils are very sensitive and important anatomical structures and should be treated properly. They should be cleansed regularly, and there are various ways of doing this. One of them, called *neti kriya*, involves cleaning the nostrils by pouring lukewarm saline water first through one nostril and then the other, allowing it to flow out the opposite side. The practice also helps prevent colds, allergies, and hayfever. Another practice is called *sutra neti*, or string cleansing. Here, a length of sterilized cotton cord, which has been blunted on one end by beeswax, is gently inserted into the nostril until it can be felt at the base of the tongue. Then you grasp this end, pulling it out through the mouth, gently moving the thread back and forth and then finally removing it, leaving the nasal passage clear. Both *kriyas* will clean out excessive mucus, open up blocked passages, and make breathing easier.

After you learn to breathe properly you will find that your thinking has become very clear. When you learn to regulate your lungs by eliminating shallowness, pauses, jerks, and noise, then you have done your work as far as cleansing the lungs is concerned.

Regulation of the breath is essential for cleansing the

lungs, but control of the breath can also be used to cleanse the pores. The yoga manuals describe many useful cleansing practices, among which are 108 kinds of baths—tub baths, herbal baths, sun baths—in fact, there are entire works devoted only to bathing. All these baths are external except one, and it is the finest of all. It is called the prana bath. For this you don't expose yourself to water, or to sun; you just sit quietly. When you bathe with water you are not cleaning the pores: an external bath can only clean the upper layers of skin. However, when you take a steam bath or sauna bath, the heat causes the pores to open and be cleansed. The prana bath is similar, but the heat is generated internally, with the help of willful breathing.

This cleansing of the pores with the help of breathing should be done only by those advanced students who have learned the method of breath retention. This exercise was developed for those students who live in caves with the desire of attaining samadhi. For them exposure to the sunlight is immaterial. The prana bath is better than the sun bath or any other bath. It is done in the accomplished posture (siddhasana) with the help of the abdominal lift, the root and throat locks, and inner retention. But it must be executed very carefully and properly or the fine tissues of the lungs will be injured. Ordinarily the preliminary exercises of breathing described earlier will be sufficient to help in cleaning the pores.

Bad odor and discoloration of the skin are symptoms of ill health, and using deodorants and unnatural soaps and lotions or medicines on the skin only hides or covers this fact. By suppressing the natural means for ridding yourself of these toxins in applying these deodorizers and other chemicals, you are only asking for trouble in the future. The extra burden of these toxins now must be taken over by the kidneys, and this will cause an excessive strain on them. The human body was designed to sweat. There is a purpose and a reason for it, and by interfering with your own cleaning system you create ill health. Besides the prana bath, cleansing the pores can be accomplished by practicing certain advanced yoga practices such as the peacock, the headstand, and bellows breathing. In fact, these provide an even better cleansing than can be accomplished by jogging or other forms of vigorous exercise.

There are certain specific cleansing exercises called *kriyas* which are described in the ancient manuals for cleaning the internal system. These techniques leave you feeling refreshed and purified of excess mucus and other wastes—and they become as important as normal bathing to the regular practitioner. The first is the upper wash, which is used to cleanse the stomach and bronchial passages. While squatting, you drink about one and a half gallons of lukewarm salted water as rapidly and as steadily as possible, and then throw it up. This is done on an empty stomach and only juices are taken afterwards. Another exercise, called *dhauti*, is designed to remove excess mucus from the esophagus and stomach. It involves swallowing a three-inch strip of sterilized white cotton cloth which is about twenty feet long. The natural gag reflex helps remove the cloth and mucus rapidly. These systems of cleansing may sound difficult at first, but once they are learned they become easy.

To modern science mucus is considered only as a secretion of the internal organs. However, to the yogis mucus is not only a secretion necessary to line the delicate internal membranes but also an excretion, a way the body rids itself of toxins. Thus excessive quantities of mucus production have always been considered by the ancients as a symptom of ill health. Many ailments of the lungs and stomach, such as asthma and certain types of indigestion, have been helped simply by practicing these washes.

Just as the regulation of the lungs and pores is important, so is regulation of the bowels and kidneys. The kidneys are the toughest filters in the body, but they need natural cleansing every day. How can the kidneys be cleaned? The ancients found that the best natural agent to clean the kidneys is whey. I have experimented with this and I agree. Whey is the liquid which is left when one separates milk to make curds. When the milk is boiling, squeeze a lemon into it, and after it curdles, strain it. The clear liquid is the whey. Whey is not very tasty, so you can use a little bit of honey in it if you like. It should not be taken hot. Used regularly, whey is a very good diuretic.

Another way to cleanse the kidneys is to make sure to drink enough liquids. Don't misunderstand: this does not mean soda pop. All carbonated beverages and liquors are unhealthy, because they irritate the intestines and leave deposits in the kidneys. I also avoid taking tap water because there are often many chemicals in it, and this too irritates the intestines and the kidneys. I take well water— but the well should be cleaned every year. Spring water is good too. Where I once lived there was a hearty stream which I drank from, but when I came down to the city I found the water packaged in bottles. No matter how wonderful water is, if it is kept bottled for prolonged periods its properties change. So I don't recommend drinking bottled water.

The best natural liquids you can take are fresh fruit and vegetable juices. A glass of fresh orange juice, cucumber juice, or lemon water taken once in the morning, or twice if necessary, is very good for cleaning the kidneys. However, it should also be remembered that when you are thirsty it is better to take pure water than to substitute with juices or bottled water.

Finally, the intestines too must be kept clean. For this, it is important to establish the habit of having a bowel movement the first thing every morning. There is an ancient practice that will help you do this. Squeeze the juice of a normal-sized fresh lemon into a glass of water which has been boiled, and add a pinch of mountain rock salt. This water should be warm, not hot, and sea salt should not be used because there is frequently sand mixed with it. Rock salt is crystallized and is much purer. The salt will draw out the waste material from the bloodstream—but too much is not good; only a little bit should be used.

Adding honey to the water will give it a little taste so that it will be easier to drink, and honey is very soothing for the intestines and good for the large colon. It is also a symbolic food. Only a bee knows how to make honey. It picks up the nectar from different places and converts it into honey. Those who are good students should be like the bee, picking up food and fragrances from different flowers and converting it into honey that is sweet to the mind and spirit.

After drinking the lemon water you should squat down, feet apart, and place one hand on each knee. Then bring the knees to the floor, one after the other, beside the foot of the opposite leg. As one leg is pushed to the floor, the opposite leg is pressed against the abdomen, creating a slight pressure on the bowels. After doing this ten or fifteen times you will feel like going to the bathroom. Drinking milk moderately every day is also very effective in emptying the bowels. Finally, if you stay on the toilet for more than five or ten minutes, there is something wrong. If you are just sitting there, thinking or reading, that is not good; it can cause hemorrhoids.

Fortunately, though, constipation is not a disease. It is caused by poor food habits, bad thinking, and a worried mind. If there is sufficient roughage in the diet there will be no problem in regulating the bowel movement. Once you have had a bowel movement you should not immediately rush for food.

The best sources of roughage are fruits, vegetables, and whole grains, not the bran that one buys at the healthfood store. Such bran is an irritant, though it may be quite effective in maintaining regularity. It is far better to obtain this roughage from whole natural foods, which contain gentler and milder forms of fiber.

Diarrhea, constipation, irregularity, and the poor functioning of the right vagus nerve (which helps digestion) can also be controlled by fasting. The Ayurvedic system says that fasting is very important for health and cleansing. But you should understand why you are fasting and should have a good reason. Some people fast for the wrong reasons, such as "If you do not listen to me, I will fast" or "I don't feel good: I should fast" or "I just want to lose ten or fifteen pounds so I'll look good." These are not good reasons. Most people do this because they have been condemning themselves. They think that they are dirty, that they have done something bad. They have not washed those impressions from their mind, and they think that by fasting they will be able to do so.

One girl told me that she had been fasting for three months. She said, "I take only one meal." This is not fasting. If it were, then I have been fasting my whole life. Many people talk about total fasting: they do not eat or drink water when they fast. That is not healthy. There is no authority in the world that recommends total fasting. When you fast you should not take solids, but you should take liquids You should take juices, like fresh orange juice, and water. You can also take some honey twice or thrice. But the finest thing to take is lemon, honey, and water.

I have fasted many times, but I do it in a very systematic way. Fasting every week is dangerous: it deteriorates the natural resistance and makes the motion of the intestines and lungs irregular. Regulating the diet by understanding the value of the food you take is much better than most of the fasting that people do. If the diet is good you don't need to fast very often. Sometimes, on special occasions and under special circumstances, it can be helpful if done under the guidance of an expert who understands the nature of the body and the purpose of the fasting.

Here I would like to mention that those who like to do fasting for reducing weight do not achieve much. Controlling the habit of overeating is easy if you learn to supply that food which is needed by the body, and particularly if you chew your food properly. Dieting does not mean fasting. At most, fasting should be done only once a month. Nothing will happen to you then if you do not eat for one day. Every three months, when the season changes, fasting for three days in a row is very important, for many illnesses catch hold of you at that time because of the climate changes.

There are many more *kriyas* or methods of cleansing mentioned in the yoga manuals. Some of them, like *dhauti*, seem crude to the modern sensibility, but students who practice and want to arrest the untimely aging process find these practices very helpful. For them, experienced teachers recommend doing yoga cleansing exercises once every three months, with fasting.

CHAPTER THREE

Nourishing

*A*LONG WITH CLEANSING techniques, the ancients stressed the importance of knowing about a balanced and nutritious diet. The body is our grossest tool and a very powerful instrument, and that which maintains the body is food. We should be practical and learn what type of food we should eat, how much food we should eat, and how much liquid we should drink. Neither overeating nor undereating is recommended. The quality of the food and the way in which it is prepared should also be understood. We should know our own capacity on all levels and regulate our diet and other activities appropriately.

There is no one diet that is perfect for all. Every person is different and unique. Each of us has a different metabolism; each requires different quantities of nutrients depending on our activity, our genetics, where we are living, and the state of our health. For example, an athlete requires much more food than a secretary, while someone who lives in the Arctic will require more vitamin D in their diet than one living in the tropics. Likewise one who is recovering from a major illness, who is thin and undernourished, requires more nourishing foods such as milk and grains, while the person who has overeaten, or has polluted their body with cigarettes or drugs, requires cleansers such as fruits. So the question of what to eat is an individual matter: each of us must decide for ourselves what and how much to eat. However, there are some general guidelines that apply to almost everyone.

First, you should not become a victim of taste. The majority of modern-day people believe in taking tasty foods without concern for their nutritional value. But it does not necessarily follow that tasty food is healthy food, nor is it essential that all healthy food be tasty. All tastes are acquired, just as other habits are. New tastes can be created by understanding that healthy food is helpful. Eating food should not become an unconscious habit like other addictions such as smoking or drinking.

Watch carefully what and how you eat. Eating large amounts of artificially flavored, highly refined junk food is dangerous to your health. Gulping down food and drink without proper chewing, or without resting between meals, or eating during stressful circumstances, leads to poor digestion. The stomach and liver will be overworked. Food will begin to ferment and putrefy in the intestines. Thus food prepared and taken in such a way works like slow poisoning. You should start by choosing a diet that consists of unprocessed, unrefined, whole foods that do not contain artificial chemicals and by eating only when the body needs nourishment.

Unfortunately, few people follow this advice. As a result of their poor food habits many people have come to use unnatural methods to force themselves to do things which should come naturally. They take a cup of tea or a glass of prune juice to go to the bathroom. To go to sleep, they take a pill. To digest food, they take a carbonated beverage. Instead of relaxing or regulating their breath to achieve a state of calm, they drink alcohol. In addition to this, over the course of a year the average person ingests more than 120 pounds of sugar, as well as several pounds of salt. Such abuse can be dangerous and even lethal. Medical research has shown that too much salt can result in high blood pressure and overtax the kidneys, and too much sugar can result in such diseases as obesity and diabetes.

On the other hand, the organic sugar in dates, honey, and fruit juices is very healthy if used in moderation. For unlike refined sugar, it is found with other nutrients in natural proportions. Nowhere in this world can one find sugar (or salt, for that matter) that is 99.9% pure—except in the supermarkets. When prepared in this form these products act more like drugs, and are even more refined than some medicines. If you eat a tablespoon of salt or a cup of sugar you will soon notice the pharmacological effects. So the next rule is to avoid using excessive quantities of salt, sugar, and other stimulants.

Most people do not know what foods they really need. They do not have a sense of what to eat. They may have a sense of when they are hungry, but then they eat anything that is easily available, without thinking about the nutritional needs of their body. People may think they are taking a proper diet, but "proper" means that which is healthy, that which does not create interference as far as one's life is concerned, and most people do not know what that is. People should be conscious of this reality, for even if they have knowledge of foods, if they don't apply it properly they will not enjoy good health. If they just had this little bit of knowledge they would lead healthier lives and become more creative, helpful, and useful. By practicing good nutrition they could protect themselves from many illnesses, maintain sound health, and even create resistance to viral diseases.

As described in the ancient manuals, food falls into two different categories: cleansers and nourishers. Fruits have more cleansing value, while vegetables, grains, legumes, and dairy products have more nourishing value. Both types of foods should be included in the normal daily diet. There should be a balance between solids and liquids. For most people this means a diet that consists of about 40% whole grains, 20% beans, 20% vegetables, 15% fruits and raw vegetable salads, and 5% dairy products. During the winter one should eat less fruit, because fruit makes one feel cooler. In the summer more fruit and raw vegetables should be taken, and the quantity of whole grains should be reduced. In this way one maintains a proper balance.

However, some people favor extremes. They become food faddists and eat only raw foods, for example. Although it is very healthy to take some raw vegetables and fruit, not all the food that makes up a balanced diet can be taken this way. Beans may be impossible to digest unless cooked, and certain vegetables contain harmful substances that are only removed by cooking. Many raw foods will irritate the linings of the intestines and cause diarrhea. In addition the intestines, appendix, and liver are not able to digest large amounts of raw food. If you were to try to live on dried fruit, for instance, your digestive mechanism would fail at some point and many undigested food particles, allowed to remain in the system for a long time, would ferment, causing excessive gas, cramps, and other gastric and intestinal problems.

It is immaterial whether you are a vegetarian or not. I am not discussing "isms" here, but healthy food values. It is true, however, that the vegetable kingdom does supply sufficient nutritional content to offer all the necessary nutrients, and for those who want to lead a spiritual life a vegetarian diet might be helpful. However, if you simply stop eating meat and substitute poor-quality foods such as candy, ice cream, or pastries, then this is not healthy either. If you want to be a vegetarian you should be certain to eat only high-quality foods.

Sunflower seeds, almonds, soybeans, dried beans and peas (dals), and some grains have sufficient protein. Indeed some seeds and nuts are as rich as meat as far as protein is concerned. There are critics who say that even if vegetarians eat the proper quantity of protein they cannot get the best quality, because there are very few non-animal proteins which are complete. This is true. The solution, however, is simply to combine a grain such as rice or wheat with a bean (dal): this creates a complete protein food that contains all the necessary amino acids in their correct ratio, without the harmful excesses of fat that are found in meats.

There are also other advantages to vegetarianism. People who are vegetarians are less likely to have constipation, hemorrhoids, and high blood pressure, as well as certain kinds of cancer and heart problems. In addition, the effects of a vegetarian diet are noticeable in old people: vegetarians have longevity of life, and in their old age they can normally think right, discuss things intelligently, and do their other duties. Many meat-eaters, on the other hand, do not show such vitality in their later years. In the animal kingdom carnivorous animals lack stamina: although they can fight fiercely, they cannot last for a long time. For instance, when the tiger and elephant fight, the tiger cannot last more than two and a half hours, but the elephant can fight for three days. The tiger is a carnivore and the elephant is a vegetarian. So it cannot be said that vegetarianism does not offer complete food value or have other benefits.

Whether you are vegetarian or non-vegetarian usually depends on your culture. Sometimes cultural habits also create problems in forming a healthy body. Such an unhealthy culture as ours needs modifications, but most human beings cling to their traditions and cultures so fanatically that they refuse to examine the cultural habits which may be making them unhealthy. Modern man calls himself civilized, but he suffers increasingly from degenerative diseases. What good is a civilization which makes one sick, weak, and incompetent?

In an attempt to slow this process of degeneration people often turn to vitamins and other nutritional supplements. They often think that these aids will be a panacea for their ills. People often ask, "How many vitamins should I take?" The ancient manuals do not even mention vitamins. However, they do speak of vitalizers such as certain juices, herbs, and other natural foods. The juice of fresh vegetables and fruits contains a very large quantity of natural vitamins and minerals, which should be taken in preference to artificial supplements. Vitamin C, for example, is readily available in the juice of fresh oranges and other fruits. These vitalizers are easy to digest in this form.

However, if the fibers of fruits and vegetables are not properly ground and pressed, the organic value of the juice will not be fully extracted. In separating the juice from the fiber, care must be taken to crush the food properly so that the juice retains the unique property of that fruit or vegetable. Being in a hurry, people often use commercial juicing machines. These give them the juice, and they drink it and think that they have taken many vitamins in this way. But many of these machines are unsuitable and are not recommended, for many of the nutrients remain unavailable. The process that should be used is one that gently presses the organic juice from the ground fibers of vegetables or fruits: in this manner all the vitamins are liberated. There are very few such machines for sale. However, no machine can be compared with our teeth, which have a powerful grip to chew the minutest fibers of food. So actually, chewing the fruits and vegetables is the best way of utilizing the properties that they contain. It should always be remembered that unchewed and unground food is not digestible, for the liver has no teeth.

Bad food and badly prepared food can affect all the nourishing organs of the body and disturb their functioning. Too many foods containing oils, for example, and too much "roasted and toasted" food or spicy food is unhealthy. It has frequently been observed that too much oily and greasy food can deteriorate the functioning of the nourishing organs. For instance, in the parts of the world where the people take in large amounts of fat and oil, many of them suffer on account of heart disease. Overcooked foods may also ultimately lead to ill health.

So you should be careful about the food you eat, being cautious not to roast, toast, and bake it too much for the sake of taste. By doing so you change the quality and also the chemical composition of the food, making it indigestible or even harmful. Furthermore it has no life, and though it feels filling, it fails to fulfill the needs of the body. In such a situation you may either overeat or lose your appetite.

However, if food is not cooked or crushed enough, it can also cause difficulties, because it will not be easily digested or processed by the liver. You can compensate for this somewhat by chewing your food very thoroughly. The purpose in eating is not merely to get the bulk of the food, but rather to take the food value from the food. Therefore the more you chew your food, the better it is for you. In addition, if you want to lose weight but don't want to curtail your meals, you should try this method: chew the food more and more and more—at least thirty-five times. If you do this you cannot overeat, and will lose weight easily. You are overeating because you are not chewing your food properly and therefore not supplying the necessary food value to the body. In other words, the body needs something, and it is not being supplied, so the body is still demanding more food.

The best method for losing weight is to eat those foods which are suitable for your own system. If the food is fresh and natural, selected and prepared properly, neither overcooked nor left undercooked, and if that food is chewed well, then you will not overeat or have a weight problem. Overeating is a very unhealthy situation and causes fat, one of the most powerful of diseases, which is also the source of many other diseases. The quantity that most people eat is more than they need, so you should watch your capacity when you eat and take a little bit less than your hunger requests.

Once you have a knowledge of food value and how to prepare food properly, you should learn how it should be eaten. It is very important to create a pleasant atmosphere before food is taken. You should not make haste or create tension before or while eating food. You should create a good mood while you are eating, for even the scientists today know that food taken while you are upset will change into poison. This has something to do with the mind, the temperament, the endocrine system, and the body as a whole. After observing and collecting data from various homes, it was found that the food served on the table may have all the necessary nutrients, but if the attitude prevailing while the family members were taking that food was not calm, or if they entered into an unpleasant discussion, they later experienced such problems as indigestion, dyspepsia, diarrhea, and constipation.

If you are angry and distressed you will not be able to create enough saliva and gastric juices: the stress, anxiety, and anger affects the glandular system and its secretions. Furthermore, under stress the intestines will become either underactive or overactive, and this too will affect the whole digestive system. Food which has not been properly digested will enter the large intestines, and there the bacteria will convert it into toxic or harmful substances. Therefore the atmosphere in which you take food is as important as the food that you take.

Never eat food, no matter how hungry you are, if you are not cheerful. Don't poison the body by making the dining table into a fighting ring. It is essential that you create a loving, pleasant attitude and atmosphere before you eat. You should start some pleasant conversation, for example. Your best friend, your greatest physician, is the cheerfulness that dwells within. So while taking food you should learn to be cheerful, for being cheerful is being creative. You should not leave this in the hands of God by saying, "God, make me cheerful"; you must create it yourself. Diversity is the essential nature of the universe, but cheerfulness is a human creation.

The ancients always said grace before eating their meals. This observance has been part of all the great traditions. This spiritual aspect of eating also has biological aspects: it makes you calm and allows the gastric juices and saliva to flow so that they can digest the food. It also helps to release tension, which allows the intestines to work properly. So saying grace or maintaining silence while relaxing and breathing deeply for a few moments before eating creates a state of harmony—a balance in the mind, body, and nervous system. Then when you eat you can relish your food. Food is not something to just be pushed in. Eating in a hurry is not healthy; it is, in fact, dangerous.

After eating it is best to rest for at least five or ten minutes by lying on the left side. By doing this the right nostril becomes active, supplying warmth and creating the necessary conditions for good digestion. This is very helpful. You can drink water half an hour after or half an hour before a meal, but drinking it while taking food is not recommended. It could be injurious to your health, for it tends to dilute and thus weaken the digestive juices. The ancients also say that it is dangerous to go to sleep right after eating. If you eat and then go to sleep immediately, your digestion will not be completed and this will affect your circulation, heart, and autonomic nervous system, and you will have bad dreams. Why should you create a situation in which you might have nightmares?

In addition, snoring can be prevented by not overeating and by learning to breathe properly. People snore for two reasons: because they are overweight, or tired. Also, you should be sure to wait for three or four hours after dinner before sexual activity, because enough time should be given to allow the body to digest the food. If you engage in sex right after eating, then the blood supply will be diverted from the digestive organs to other parts of the body, and digestion will be incomplete.

It is healthy to take juices, fruit, and other foods in small quantities several times a day rather than overeating or having a large, heavy meal at one time. For lack of time many businessmen and busy people take dinner late in the day. It becomes heavy for the system and is not digested in time before sleeping. The evening meal should be very light. Midnight meals disturb the body.

Food taken at fixed hours also counts a lot. I collected data especially from bar attendants who work late at night and air hostesses who travel on international flights. Their digestive systems are always irregular, and many of the hostesses reported to me that their menstrual period became irregular when they led an irregular life. Food and sleep influence the body. If food is taken on time, the system is regulated because of the regular habit. Irregularly taken meals during odd hours create acidity in the system. Similarly there are countless other diseases which are acquired by irregular eaters.

If you take these little precautions and practice these methods you can avoid dyspepsia and other diseases and enjoy good health. These are the things that everyone should understand; they comprise the difference between human beings and animals. If a person has a dish before them, they can say, "I'm not eating; it is not healthy for me." If their doctor says not to eat something, that person won't eat it, no matter how delicious the dish might be. But animals and young children cannot do this; they do not have enough sense or training. Sensible people, on the other hand, understand when they are eating improperly or getting too attached to food, and then they change their patterns The ancients cooked their food and ate it as an offering to God who created it for them, his instruments. It is important to remain healthy to be the instrument of the Lord and do one's duties selflessly. For those who understand the secret of life, their day-to-day life becomes an act of worship.

CHAPTER FOUR

Exercise

*T*HE TWO DIFFERENT KINDS of physical exercise essential to good health are stretching exercises (such as the yoga postures) and aerobic exercises (such as jogging). Both are very beneficial for cleansing, relaxing, and revitalizing the body and for helping it function properly.

Although quite different, they complement each other. The postures are relaxed, slow, and gentle. They provide systematic stretching to all the muscles and joints of the body, and massage the glands and organs. Aerobic exercise is active and stimulates the heart, lungs, and muscles. Both kinds are necessary; each has unique effects which the other cannot produce. But they must be practiced regularly, carefully, and in the correct manner in order to attain the desired effect. Doing either beyond your capacity does more harm than good.

These days body therapies like massage, chiropractic, Rolfing, bioenergetics, and reflexology are very popular. They all have specific benefits, but are limited in two respects: you need to rely on a therapist to provide the treatment, and the effects tend to be short-lived unless you return again and again for more treatments. The yoga postures, on the other hand, are perfected gradually. This encourages self-reliance, and as you practice, observing your physical and emotional reactions, you will begin to notice definite positive changes in both body and mind.

An obvious effect of the yoga postures comes from the stretch and stimulation they give to the muscles, ligaments, and joints. This restores elasticity and tone to the body so that it eventually regains its natural shape. In addition, the yoga postures stimulate circulation, revitalizing the internal viscera, the brain, and the nervous system. Your respiratory system performs more efficiently when you do the postures, for greater amounts of oxygen can then enter the system and more toxins can be eliminated. All the internal organs are massaged and toned, improving not only digestion but also bowel and kidney function. The endocrine system is stimulated and regulated to a fine balance. The postures increase resistance to fatigue and relieve tension. You learn how to relax, allowing the systems of the body to function properly. So the postures are a good, gentle tonic for the entire personality, making you feel healthy and full of energy. Excess weight is also reduced; the body becomes supple, and you move with greater grace and ease. The complexion glows, the eyes shine.

By practicing the postures regularly you gain control of the body and are able to maintain a steady, comfortable pose for increasingly greater lengths of time. You then begin to observe the finer functions of breath and mind, for only when the body is still can you turn within and begin to know yourself.

The basic goals of the yoga postures are to maintain a healthy body and gain peace of mind. Yoga texts tell us that many physical complaints come about in the following way: a psychological disturbance leads to a functional impairment, which in turn is reflected in irregularities in the breathing patterns; if this process continues it can lead to actual cellular damage and manifest itself in a structural alteration. The yoga postures work first to correct the structural alteration and can be used as an effective therapy (particularly in the early stages) in reversing the above process. Then breath-awareness and various breathing exercises can be useful in eliminating the irregularities which have developed in the breathing patterns. They can thereby help resolve the psychological disturbance which created the alteration in the first place. Thus, changes brought about through the practice of postures are not sudden or dramatic; they are deep and permanent.

At first the postures may seem awkward, but they have been systematically developed for centuries, through direct experience and observation, to calm, balance, and regulate the systems of the body. When done properly and patiently at a regular time and place one enjoys them, and they become a habit which brings a deep sense of calmness and much satisfaction.

There are over three thousand yoga postures, but only a few are basic. Among them are the cobra, boat, bow, plow, shoulderstand, fish, forward bend, spinal twist, headstand, and stomach lift. The yogis lived close to nature and keenly observed their fellow creatures. Consequently many of the postures (for example the cobra, locust, fish, scorpion, frog) are based on certain unique characteristics a particular animal displays. The postures are both natural and universal in nature and can be practiced by most people if they begin gradually, under the guidance of a competent teacher. It is not true that you cannot do them because it is not a part of your heritage: anyone who wants to practice the postures can do so within their own capacity. But you should never strain or push for immediate results;

doing so could cause injury and pain.

Practice in a quiet place, comfortably warm and free from drafts, where you can spread a blanket to lie on. Do the postures after bathing, in loose clothing. Stomach, bladder, and bowels should be empty. Perform the postures systematically, with control and awareness, a calm mind, and an attitude of respect. The mind remains passively alert and watchful; only those parts of the body needed to hold the pose should be tensed.

It is best to begin with some gentle warm-up stretches such as joints and glands exercises. Start with the easier postures and work up to the more difficult ones. Most of the poses are complementary and should be done in a proper sequence with a short rest between each. Performing them in the morning prepares the body and mind for the activities of the day. Performing them at night soothes the nerves and helps one to relax. Since the body is more flexible at night the postures are more easily done then, but morning practice sets a wonderful tone for the entire day. So fit them in according to your own schedule and temperament.

In addition to the postures you can also practice dynamic aerobic exercises. Jogging is very good for this. Jogging is popular nowadays, but there is much misunderstanding about the proper way to perform it, and many people have harmed themselves by doing it incorrectly. Some people force themselves, pushing and straining and trying to do too much too soon. You should always prepare yourself first and work within your comfortable capacity. You should enjoy jogging; it should not be a form of self-torture.

Jogging has been shown to be effective in reducing depression and major psychoses as well as in decreasing anxiety. It appears to be at least as effective as psychotherapy or tranquilizers with borderline schizophrenics, and it works as well as group psychotherapy with neurotics. It increases mental concentration and clarity, and it makes one alert and energetic. Those who jog are less affected by stressful situations than those who do not, and they respond to them less, physically and emotionally, because they do not secrete as many excitory hormones when under sudden shock or ongoing pressure. Those who jog sleep less than most and more soundly, and since they are not drowsy when they are awake, they do not need to rely on coffee, cigarettes, or sleeping pills in order to work or relax. Jogging gives one a natural and healthy outlet for expressing the physiological reactions of the fight-or-flight response to threatening situations.

So much of modern life is full of stress that if you do not have a way to overcome the resulting tension or to express it beneficially, then you keep it inside. That can make you sick; it is one of the reasons people have ulcers, heart attacks, headaches, and upsetting emotions. They do not know how to live in the world and yet remain centered and calm within, above the rush and roar of daily life. Jogging can definitely help you in this way, and it does this by making some specific changes in the body.

First of all, it helps your lungs operate more efficiently, strengthening the muscles around them, making them stronger, increasing their vital capacity, decreasing their residual volume, and opening up previously unused space. Circulation is increased as the networks of blood vessels open up to nourish and cleanse the body. The heart is strengthened and toned, making it very healthy; in fact, it is actually enlarged, thus increasing its efficiency. The resting heart rate is decreased through jogging, as is the heart rate required for any given level of exertion. This happens because the heart pumps more blood with each stroke; it thus needs to beat less frequently, thereby conserving energy.

Through jogging the muscles increase in tone and strength, so you move with greater speed, endurance, flexibility, and grace. Jogging burns calories (one hundred calories per mile), but more important, it resets the appetite mechanism in the brain, so you eat less and lose weight. In addition, less acid than usual is secreted in the stomachs of joggers, thus decreasing the possibility of ulcers. Jogging also acts as a natural cathartic, so that the bowels of joggers are usually regular, and constipation is rare. Jogging also helps to normalize diabetes, hypoglycemia, and other blood-sugar problems. It purifies the entire system, aiding the elimination of wastes from the bowels, bladder, pores, mucus membranes, lungs, and the cells themselves. Through jogging the pain threshold is modified, so you are less distracted by bodily discomfort. Thus the whole body functions more smoothly and efficiently when you jog, and the mind and emotions are calmed.

To begin jogging, it is best to dress warmly in absorbent clothes such as cotton sweatsuits, but any loose clothing will do. Keeping the body warm helps the cleansing process by increasing sweating. Any comfortable running shoe is good, but if you run on the pavement the shoe should be well-cushioned. Running on the earth is better, but extra caution must be taken to avoid stumbling and injuring yourself. Before jogging it is very important to stretch the muscles and to practice some deep breathing exercises.

Jogging can be slow, regular, and steady, so you can go for a long time without tiring. Done this way it is gentle but very effective, and it will not harm the body. Proper breathing for jogging is always diaphragmatic, and you should breathe through your nose, exhaling for twice as long as you inhale. Exhalations should be complete, so all the toxins are eliminated from the system.

It is helpful to listen to the sound of the air going out over the soft palate and through the nostrils while you concentrate on exhaling completely. A good way to set the proper pace for jogging is by observing your need for air: if you cannot get enough breath through your nose, then you are going too fast and straining, and you should pull back. It is possible to go to almost your maximum capacity while you are still breathing through your nose. If you feel that you cannot get enough air, you are exceeding your limit. If that happens you should break your jog and walk until you catch your breath. You should jog comfortably at about three-quarters of your capacity.

Jogging on the balls of your feet is the best way to go for these slow jogs. This keeps the movement light and flowing and cushions the feet, ankles, shins, knees, and hips, protecting them from injury due to a harsh impact. Landing on the toes also increases the massaging and stimulating effects of jogging.

Do not let your mouth hang open or your arms flop when you jog. Remember that you are breathing through your nose. Keep your lips together. Gently hold your arms up close to your chest, with your loose fists rotating about your chest as you move, and keep your elbows close to your body. Be sure to keep your shoulders relaxed and your head up. Keep your spine straight, your whole body relaxed, and let the abdomen move freely in and out as you breathe.

Always jog with full concentration, particularly on the breathing, and enjoy the process. This will bring a feeling of clarity, peace, and energy, for the muscles are relaxed, the oxygen in the lungs and bloodstream is flowing freely, and the mind has calmed down. But this is not the same as meditation. In jogging the body is active, and so the mind is active, but in meditation both are still.

You should take care when you are jogging downhill, slowing down and landing gently so that you do not injure your knees or feet. Jogging itself should be rhythmic and natural. I have watched the faces of some joggers who look as if they were in agony as they pound down the street. This is not the way. The movement should be smooth and graceful. You should enjoy it, and you should always let up if you are in pain. Do not ignore the pain; learn from it so you can discover the proper way to jog. Experiment until you find a way that is not painful to you. Your body will direct you to the natural way if you do not force it. Be kind but disciplined, gentle but firm.

There are several variations to jogging that give one special benefits. A very good one is the twisting jog. Here, the torso and arms twist from side to side in rhythm with the pace. The arms create momentum as they swing, and the level at which the hands are held helps determine the point of the twist. This twisting and turning invigorates the spinal nerves and massages the viscera. Another variation is jogging with the arms raised high overhead with the hands folded. This lifts and expands the chest so that more fresh air can flow through the lungs, and it gives a good stretch to the arms, chest, and abdomen. A third style is to lift the knees high and to kick the heels toward the buttocks as you jog. This helps the knee joints and exerts more effort.

When you have finished jogging do not stop abruptly; slow down gradually or you will stiffen. If you have been breathing properly, profuse sweating may occur, and this will cleanse the entire system. You should avoid taking a bath or shower until at least half an hour after jogging, however, because it may shock the system, and the pores should be given time to keep the sweat flowing. You should keep warm during this time.

It is good to stretch again after jogging to avoid cramps

or sore muscles. The yoga postures are best for this. You can do them either before or after jogging, or both. Jogging after postures leaves you loose and stimulated; jogging before postures leaves you calm and balanced for the day. But if all you can do is jog, then do it. Do the postures at another time.

You will be more likely to jog regularly if you make it a part of your daily schedule. Then it becomes a habit which you accept and which the body automatically prepares for. In this way unconscious resistance is lessened. If you are obese, older, or very out of shape you should begin by walking before you jog. You can get yourself started by taking the easiest step in that direction. Just stop what you are doing and go outside when it is time. If you do not want to change clothes, then jog in what you are already wearing. If you feel too tired to jog, then just walk, and soon you can pick up the pace. Often you will find that you are not as tired as you thought you were. But don't set rigid limits for yourself. If you have determined to go for fifteen mintues and feel too tired to continue after ten, then stop. Let your body guide you. You should gain energy from jogging, not lose it. Do not push, but also do not be lazy. After several weeks of daily practice, jogging will become a habit.

At dawn the air has a special quality, and it is very good to jog then. Late afternoon, when your energy may be low, is another good time to jog. When you are feeling low already is another good time, because jogging will reset the metabolism and invigorate you. It is also hardest to get going then, so just form the habit, and it will be easier to do it. Never jog on a full stomach, however; let at least several hours go by after a meal.

Jogging out of doors is better than doing it inside, but jogging inside, or even jogging in place, is better than not doing it at all. Jogging twice a day is an excellent practice.

It need not take longer than fifteen minutes to gain the benefits. One hundred breaths is a good run, and so is five hundred steps at a comfortable, loose pace. Three miles a day is a good goal to work toward. Long, fast jogs are not as effective as regularly practiced slower and shorter ones for attaining all the physical and emotional benefits possible.

In the early stages jogging may be difficult, since you cannot do as much as you would like to, but growth occurs in plateaus, and one day you will suddenly be able to do much more than you could before if you do not set your progress back by giving up or by pushing too much. Do not do either, for jogging is a powerful practice which creates overall well-being and a sound inner environment for spiritual development. It is the perfect complement to the yoga postures.

Women can do all of these exercises just as men can, but they should refrain from performing them during menstruation, the last five or six months of pregnancy, and the first six weeks or so after delivery. Women should view the first few days of the menstrual cycle as an opportunity to rest and practice relaxation, diaphragmatic and alternate nostril breathing, meditation, and inspirational reading rather than doing any strenuous exercise. The body is going through a natural cleansing process at this time, and it is not healthy to divert energy away from the places it is needed. This is not a sexist bias; it is a physiological reality. Practicing postures or jogging at this time could cause cramps and excess bleeding. Practiced at other times, however, the exercises create a strong and regular constitution which makes the so-called female problems less of a problem: less discomfort and fewer irregularities are experienced during periods, and menstrual disorders are corrected.

Pregnancy and deliveries are also made easier if one has been practicing the postures regularly. Some simple standing, seated, squatting, and reclining postures which do not affect the abdomen can be continued during menstruation, pregnancy, and postpartum adjustment, but the inverted, backward-bending, and forward-bending postures are not recommended. The squatting posture can help decrease discomfort from cramps during menstruation. After the fourth month of pregnancy women should cease all postures except for a few simple stretching exercises. Any postures involving the pelvic area can be dangerous to the unborn child. Women who want to begin the yoga postures for the first time should wait until six months after delivery to start.

The most beneficial posture for an expectant mother is the relaxation pose, which should be practiced extensively along with diaphragmatic breathing. Pregnant women should not jog at all, but regular walking is very good. When jogging, women should protect their breasts, wearing garments that support them firmly or holding them still by folding their arms underneath them. Women should be especially careful to jog on the balls of their feet in order to land gently and prevent displacement of the uterus. Jogging seems to be an especially beneficial practice for women, since they seem to be prone to the complaints it corrects and also because they frequently do not engage in other forms of physical activity.

Children are naturally flexible and eager to play, stretch, and run. They enjoy their bodies and love to learn new ways to experience them. In a household where the yoga postures and jogging are practiced, the children will pick them up by watching their parents; otherwise they can be taught a simple program of postures by age seven or nine. But since they have shorter attention spans and lack the muscle strength and control of adults, the length of time they hold the postures should be shorter, and they should not be forced to go beyond their limitations. Care should be taken in teaching the inverted postures to children, since their bones and muscles are not fully developed and they cannot safely support their own weight.

Prolonged practice of the shoulderstand is not advised for prepubescents, because of its stimulating effects on the thyroid gland, which regulates growth. Children under twelve can perform the cobra, half locust, bow, forward bend, plow, and yoga mudra without harm, but it would be best to avoid the headstand, peacock, stomach lift, and other difficult practices until age twelve or puberty. Adolescence is a good time to begin the practice of the yoga postures, but it is not so essential in childhood.

Jogging is very good for children. Although they generally run and play a great deal, a surprising number are not in good shape, because they do not take part in regular exercise. Jogging gives them a good way to do this. It also helps them release built-up energy and provides a chance for the entire family to do something together. Jogging is good for children who are not very skillful at team sports or who dislike competition. It is a healthy activity and can help children feel better about themselves at the same time. Children should be careful, however, not to overexert themselves or exercise without paying attention to their motions.

These exercises will give children strength, endurance, agility, and coordination, and will also prevent many diseases while improving their state of mind. It has also been found that the mental functioning of children can be increased by enlarging their intake of oxygen through correct deep breathing—and breathing is improved by both postures and jogging. Good habits formed in childhood shape the life of the adult to be.

Advanced age, however, is not a barrier to beginning, or practicing, the yoga postures if it is done with care. It is never too late to begin, or resume, these exercises, and their benefits are always available. The postures are beginning to be taught in nursing homes, and the elderly enjoy practicing them gently and experiencing their effects.

Older people need not merely await degeneration and death. They can use their time to become healthier than they ever were—but they should begin with gentle stretching exercises, and they should always be careful not to extend beyond their comfortable capacity. They can benefit a great deal from the yoga postures, since these postures have a beneficial effect on many common ailments of old age, such as hypertension, stroke, diabetes, insomnia, arthritis, digestive disorders, constipation, and chronic aches and pains. Stiff joints, brittle bones, and fragile ligaments and muscles should be protected by cautious awareness, but within these limits the elderly can increase their enjoyment of life with a program of these stretches.

The same is true of jogging if the older person begins gradually, with a regular program of daily walking. The pace can eventually become faster and the distance longer until it is comfortable to do a slow jog once or twice a day. This is very good for regulating and rejuvenating the entire system. Weak and infirm people in nursing homes have become healthy, lively, and happy because they have taken up exercise programs consisting of jogging and postures. The quality of their lives can definitely be improved so that they look forward to surviving longer. Illness often follows inactivity and depression, but it can be removed with exercise and a sense of purpose and well-being. There are many marathon runners who are in their seventies. Age is no excuse to avoid taking responsibility for your health.

A measure of vitality, awareness, and peace is thus available to all who seek it, and a good way to start is to get the body in a healthy condition through exercise. Only when you are healthy and strong can the mind, will, and emotions be trained, and this is essential for spiritual growth.

CHAPTER FIVE

Being Still

T IS ONLY AFTER you have learned to take care of the body that you can tread the path of inner life. Proper cleansing, nourishing, and exercise are the prerequisites for the next step in the cultivation of health. This step is called being still. It is very important and, if you study it systematically, not very difficult. Once you have prepared the body, it is essential that you learn to sit quietly. Even if you eat the best diet, if you do not know how to be still your mind will not yet be under your control. The most magnificent sports car, if it is driven recklessly, will soon be destroyed: so it is also with the human being. A strong body willed by a reckless mind leads to restlessness and ill health. You should become aware of the integration of the mind and body, for the mind and body have such a close relationship that the body can disturb the mind: if the body is in a state of pain or disease, then the mind will also be ill at ease. Likewise, a restless mind creates a tense and nervous body.

It should be remembered, however, that in general the mind rules the body. The mind moves first, and then the body follows. So your body language is totally dependent on your mental functions. Try this and see. Try to raise your arm without first thinking about it. It cannot be done. In order to raise the arm you must first think "Arm, raise," and then send this message through the nervous system from the brain to the arm. The arm will not move until the mind tells it to do so.

Furthermore, just as the mind sends messages to the body, the body is continually sending messages to the mind—"This chair is hard; this posture causes a pain in the back," and so on. When the mind is constantly being badgered by all these body messages it becomes very active, agitated, and dissipated trying to integrate all the data. It cannot remain calm.

Therefore in order to learn to be still you must first quiet the chatter coming from the body. This begins by learning the art of sitting. By developing a steady, comfortable position you free yourself from the distractions of the body and are able to attend to the mind. For if your body is not steady your mind cannot be still; if you put your body into an uncomfortable position it will become a constant source of distraction. In addition, if you sit in a certain position for a week and then change to another position the next week, your mental attitude will change as well. So choosing a position in which you can be still is very important.

The Bible talks about the importance of stillness: "Be still, and know that I am God." (Psalm 46:10) If you learn this, then that godly part in you will reveal itself. But for that godly part to be revealed without being still is not possible. So you should direct your voluntary and conscious effort to learning how to be still. If you just learn this, there will be no problem. In the beginning this means not moving at all. Later, once you learn what stillness is, you will be able to move the body, to act and live in the world, yet remain still. Calmness, stillness, and a one-pointed mind are identical; when this is realized, it becomes possible to create them at all times. In other words, true stillness does not merely mean the absence of movement: it means having equanimity, and then performing your actions responsibly; it means attending effortlessly to your duties without being unduly affected by external circumstances.

To achieve this goal requires, first of all, self-discipline. Whereas all the activities of animals are governed by nature, that is not the case with human beings. Human actions are governed by human desires, and these can be controlled only through self-discipline.

Many people are afraid of the word "discipline," for discipline when imposed by others is definitely frightening. But self-accepted discipline helps keep the body healthy and the mind sound. Discipline really means regulating habits, and habits are the basis of human character. You spend your whole life identifying with your personality, with your character. But who built it? God? Nature? No. Your own habits have woven a character for you, and their pattern makes up your personality. Your habits are deep-rooted in motivation. You can strengthen these habits, or you can change them.

If you really want to change and understand how habits are formed, then you will come to know that there are simple practices for doing this. With time, and with the help of these laws, you can systematically bring about that inner transformation which is called *samyama* in the ancient texts. You cannot change your face or other external forms and shapes, but you can completely transform your internal states. Today you might condemn yourself and feel bad about yourself because of your habits, but tomorrow you can completely transform yourself and come in touch with your inner potentials for creativity, happiness, and truth.

Self-discipline can be achieved only through the conscious directing of your will. Will is a very powerful tool for making you successful—and willpower is created by a one-pointed and concentrated mind. The more your mind is dissipated, the more willpower weakens. It is not easy to control the totality of the mind, for the mind is vast. In fact the ancient scriptures say "Vastest of all is the mind." There is only one thing that is vaster than the mind, and that is the center of consciousness. But that portion of the mind which you use in your daily life can be brought under control very easily if you learn and practice a systematic approach.

The first thing to learn is regularity, or consistency in your practice. To do this you should form the habit of sitting quietly once or twice every day. For learning to be still it is important to find a comfortable and steady pose, either on a chair or on the floor. Steadiness comes when you keep your head, neck, and trunk in a straight line. For a few days this might create a little bit of uneasiness, but gradual and gentle practice will help you in sitting steadily and comfortably. Again, overdoing this is not at all recommended. It is better to sit correctly for five minutes twice a day than to sit once a week for an hour.

In trying to find a position in which to sit, many people who have read Eastern books begin with difficult postures, such as *padmasana* (the lotus pose) and *siddhasana* (the accomplished pose), without first making their body supple. By doing this you can strain the knees and cause pain, discomfort, and even physical injury. You will be disturbed by the discomfort and will not achieve stillness. Instead of doing this you should sit in any easy pose that makes you comfortable and straight.

Then you can learn to be physically steady. It is important to keep the head, neck, and trunk straight, because if you are sitting crooked or are slumping over you are not allowing the spinal cord to be aligned correctly. Then the three sensitive channels there—the central canal in the middle, and the sympathetic and parasympathetic cords on either side—cannot function properly. When the body is still you should not be tense: any tension will be reflected in your muscles and nervous system. Your whole body structure, the way you are sitting, needs to form a steadiness for you.

Practicing one posture every day at the same time is very important. So you should practice a posture in which you are comfortable and steady. One posture that should not be used for this process is the corpse pose. This pose, done by lying on the back with the legs and hands at the sides slightly away from the body, does induce deep relaxation and is very comfortable, but it is not considered steady. By practicing this pose, however, you can learn to ease physical tension.

Releasing physical tension is very important, because muscle tension can create havoc in your body, affecting the heart, brain, liver, and digestive system. In learning to relax you should lie down on the back with the legs about eighteen inches apart, the hands on the abdomen, and if the surface is hard, a soft pillow cushioning the head. Then systematically survey the body from head to toe and back, locating the tension points and mentally releasing them. Once you understand your own mental capacity you will be able to be successful in doing this within a few days' time.

It is very important that you not use autosuggestion, but rather observe the movement of the diaphragm and then breathe gently and deeply according to your comfortable capacity. Making the body still and then making the flow of the breath serene and deep will help in relaxing the nervous system and releasing the tension from the set of muscles that is governed by the autonomic nervous system. This relaxation exercise should not be practiced for more than ten minutes; otherwise you might fall asleep. After five minutes you should voluntarily create tension all over the body, release it, survey the body again, and watch the slow, deep flow of the breath.

By practicing this exercise regularly you will reap many benefits: blood pressure will be lowered; the heart, liver, and digestive organs will function more effectively; you will have less tension, more strength and energy, and greater vitality. Simply by doing the corpse posture along with deep abdominal breathing increases longevity and fosters health.

One final reminder regarding regularity is that you should choose a specific time and consistently use that time to practice sitting. The best time is either early in the morning or in the evening. However, any time is fine as long as you will not be bothered by other duties, interruptions, or distractions. Regulating your habits by being punctual in practice is important because it is necessary to counteract the pressure of bad habits which keep the body under stress. A body which remains constantly under the influence of such habits will always be unhealthy.

The second point to understand and observe in learning to be still is that it is necessary to cultivate patience with yourself. Suppose you want to sit calmly—but since you have never learned to do so you can sit for only two minutes before your mind starts jumping about. You change your posture, try again to be still—and then change your posture again. You should accept this. Failure is the pillar of success—provided you take advantage of the situation and learn from it. You should observe your capacity and go slowly. The first day two minutes is sufficient. It is said in the scriptures that if you can sit still, straight, and comfortably with a perfectly one-pointed mind for just ten minutes, you can attain samadhi. So it is best to increase your capacity slowly and gradually and to learn to be patient with yourself.

Patience is a great virtue—but what does it mean? It does not mean being lazy, nor does it mean an absence of effort or the failure to plan ahead. Being patient means being observant. Once you learn to be patient you will not condemn yourself for problems with your thinking process. Patience is like standing on the bank of the river of life just waiting for your ship to return. There is a flow. You do not repeat that which is done; you do not see that which is not yet done. You are patiently waiting to see the fruits of your deeds, being content with doing your best and thus making wise decisions for the future.

So you should learn to be patient with yourself. You know yourself better than anybody else. That part of your personality which has never been exposed to others you yourself know—for you always remains in touch with that part of yourself which is not pleasant. Many people start identifying themselves with that part of their personalities and start condemning themselves. They do something one day, and the next day start condemning themselves for it. If the world does not praise them, if people do not appreciate them, they blame themselves. They are not aware of the innate source of strength within themselves. They should learn to appreciate and admire that part in them which is helping them, leading them. No matter how much they condemn themselves, no matter how bad they think they are—and even if the whole world says they are bad—still there are certain qualities in them which are very special and which make them unique. They should learn to admire those parts.

If the first step in developing stillness is making it into a daily habit, and the second is being patient with yourself, then the third is practicing constant observation. You should learn to observe your capacity. Although you may like to practice sitting, sometimes in the beginning of developing this habit the mind will say "What am I doing? This is silly. Nobody in our culture does this. Why should I be still? This is a foolish idea. Why don't I just get up and have a Coke?" But no matter what culture or religion you come from, you should learn to be still for the sake of your health.

If you really follow these principles there will be no problem. You should understand from the very beginning that stillness is essential, because you cannot attain meditation until you can be still. Whenever you are attentive you have to be still: this is a principle. You cannot properly examine an object when in motion.

Physical stillness, however, does not mean mental stillness. When you learn to still the body, something else becomes more active. To make your body still means to make your mind active: when you finally begin calming down your conscious mind you find that the unconscious mind is activated, rushing in with memories, thoughts, and feelings, many of which were previously suppressed.

In the process of meditation you first contact the conscious part of your mind and learn of body-mind interaction. The conscious mind is that which you use in your daily life during the waking state. By sitting in a particular place, using the same posture, holding the head, neck, and trunk straight, observing your thoughts as they emerge, you are slowly able to begin to contact and calm the conscious mind and body. At this stage, you should pay attention to the body tremors and muscle tension, consciously releasing any muscular tightness that is perceived. Later, as the conscious mind and the body begin to rest, the unconscious mind becomes active and emerges into awareness.

In the beginning you should not overdo your practice. It is your ambitious mind that says you should try to do it for a long time, that you can sit for half an hour. This is a waste of time. Looking at your watch to see how many minutes you have practiced is not helpful. You shouldn't try to show that you are a great yogi. You have to be great from within. Gradually, in a few months if you practice, you can learn to be still for a longer time—but there is no use in wasting time absentmindedly daydreaming and hallucinating various images and calling it meditation.

When you sit to meditate, your memory becomes more active. You recall what you have done in the past, who has been good to you, who has been bad to you, who has been your friend, who has been your enemy. Sometimes the unconscious brings forward one of the impressions from the bed of your memory that makes you either happy or unhappy, and you forget that you are sitting for meditation, allowing yourself to be completely carried away by that thought-form. Involvement with thought-forms in this way is not meditating, it is daydreaming. It is a waste of energy, because it actually strengthens that part of the mind that is uncontrolled. So in order to learn the process of being still you must gain control over the conscious mind.

At first, when the mind is flying here and there, it will be very helpful to practice breath-awareness. This is very important, for the breath is quite closely related to the conscious mind. They are interdependent: when the breath stops, the conscious mind fails, and that is called death. You can train and regulate the mind by being aware of your breathing, for breathing is the lamp that lights the path to increased awareness. By simply learning to observe the breathing process you can reach a deep state of meditation.

However, the first few days this will be an obstacle,

because you are trying to bring your conscious mind under control, whereas previously it had been controlling you. It will resist and will not want to listen. As you start to control it, however, it will change completely. When you first begin you may notice while inhaling that suddenly the inhalation breaks and you feel as if you are suffocating or not able to catch your breath: if you continue to pay attention to the breath and nothing else, this feeling will soon disappear. Let the mind be aware of the breath and watch how it flows. If you can do this for three minutes—only three minutes without any diversion—it will bring good results.

Besides observing the breath you should also be aware of the sensitivity of the nervous system. Some people mistake sensitivity for psychic ability, but that is an error. I once had an experience that illustrates this point:

When I was a child living in Kalipur on the border between Tibet and India I studied kung fu. I had been taught not to harm, hurt, or kill anyone, and I became very passive, because I did not understand the principle of nonviolence properly. If an animal charged me, I would not defend myself. So I was sent to a kung fu teacher who was over ninety years old. This old man had been blind from birth—but if I moved my finger in a circle he would say, "You are making a circle"; if I shook it he would say, "Now you are shaking your finger." I suspected that he could really see and that he knew some trick to make himself appear blind—but when I asked him how he could do these things and told him of my suspicion, he showed me his empty eye sockets. I was amazed, but even then I thought "There is some trick here. He knows how to turn his eyeballs in a different way." I was that skeptical.

One day he said, "Come over here. I am going to show you that I see everything not through my eyes, but through my sensitivity. I want ten of you to come at me with sticks and try your best to hit me. I won't have a stick myself."

I said, "I won't do it because you are a blind man." He replied, "You are taking useless pity on me for being blind. I am not. My nervous system is so active and sensitive that I can perceive any sound vibrations that happen near me better than you can. I can see things through my nervous system; I don't need eyes."

Then some of the students who knew him well started to attack him. He was in the center of a circle of ten people and quietly went through a gap in the circle, leaving the students hitting each other. He started laughing and said, "Do it again."

The second time, he snatched somebody's stick and started fighting with everybody. Nobody could hurt him. He was so sensitive to the things going on around him that he checked any move that was made. Through discipline and will this man had developed his nervous sensitivity to a very high degree. He was able to see without sight.

Normally when you look at something the sensation is carried by the optic nerve to the brain and then is distributed to the related parts of the body. The nervous system lies between the brain and the body. The body is actually like a house, and the nervous system is a large network of electrical wires. The brain is like a lightbulb, and the mind is the energy which constantly flows through that network which is the nervous system. If the house is not properly looked after, all its electrical potential will be of no use. Likewise, if you have a wonderful mind but your brain is damaged, then your energy will not be used properly. Even if your brain and mind are both very good, if your nervous system is defective then your potential will not be realized.

All living creatures possess a nervous system, but each differs in its degree of sensitivity. For example if a plant is cut, tears do not flow down its leaves: though it has a nervous system of sorts, it is not very evolved. If you cut or hurt your foot, however, you will cry immediately, and tears will roll down from your eyes: you have an active nervous system. Nervous sensitivity is not just a physical trait; it is also a mental and emotional one. This actively working nervous system in human beings is a gift in the cycle of evolution, and we should take advantage of it by developing it properly.

Many people are insensitive in their relationships, because they don't understand how to cultivate the sensitivity within them. But one's emotional life is totally dependent on this sensitivity. Sensitivity is part of awareness. Many times when people talk they say "I am aware of [this, that, or the other]"—they are talking about certain facts, about being aware of something physical, something quite obvious. Yet despite being sensitive to these external or superficial matters, many people remain oblivious to what is happening within.

This changes when a person begins to meditate. During the early stages of meditation they can become very aware and very sensitive to the things they have done in the past, and may feel guilty or unhappy about them. Rather than accept these feelings most people resist them, for they do not know how to forgive themselves. They blame themselves. They have formed this habit, and apply it to others too. So if somebody has done something which they don't like, they don't forgive them, either. Gradually they have made themselves insensitive to the positive things in themselves and in others; they see only the negative.

You should learn to forgive by doing it occasionally whether it is contrary to your desires or not. If you have committed a mistake you should accept the fact that a mistake is only a mistake. You should not repeat it, but should not condemn your personality for it. In this way you can increase your ability to be sensitive.

If you do not appreciate and accept yourself, it is because you have been doing negative meditation. This has made you what you are today. Worry is one form of negative meditation, and it can become a deep-seated unconscious habit. You can create many diseases through your own mind—and you can heal yourself through this same mind. So you should learn to give yourself positive feedback: "I am all right. The life-force is here in me. Why am I condemning myself? Why am I hurting myself?" That mind which has the power to create guilt feelings and many diseases also has the power to heal, for it is completely controlled by the thinking process. Just learn that the mind is creating diseases, and try to heal them instead.

Meditation is very powerful and therapeutic. There could not be anything more powerful than meditation. I learned this lesson once when I was a boy. I fell down the mountainside and injured my right knee. A large, persistent lump developed there. One of the swamis said, "You can dissolve that lump with your mind."

I said, "I don't want that lump, and yet it is still there."

He said, "You don't want yourself to be a bad boy—and yet you are a bad boy. What do you mean by 'want'? Want is not powerful: you want yourself to be good, and still you are not; you want that lump to dissolve, and still it does not. So wanting has nothing to do with it. Learn to meditate. In meditation a one-pointed mind is developed, and this creates a dynamic will. Willpower is a greater and deeper strength than wanting."

I told him, "You do meditation. If you think your mind is very powerful, then why don't you just help me and dissolve this lump?"

He agreed and said that he would. He told me to sit

down at such and such a time and in one week the lump would be gone. He said, "I could dissolve it right now, but I want you to become aware of the process and learn." In exactly one week the lump disappeared. I could not find a trace of it.

The first principle of learning to be still is regular practice; the second is patience; the third is observation; and the fourth is analysis. It is true that you must understand yourself from within to attain a state of perfection—but analysis is not sufficient to transform the personality. After analysis comes the discrimination to make a proper decision. You should never determine to do something unless you have explored all the consequences and chosen the best alternative for your development. This principle of choosing the best alternative is called discrimination, and is the fifth principle for developing control of the mind.

The reason you experience failure is that you do not know how to make decisions at the right time and place. Your faculty of discrimination cannot decide in time, because there is no strength behind it. One Urdu poem says "When I was young I had strength, but no wisdom. Now that I am old I have wisdom, but no strength." When you do not know how to decide things in time, there is a misuse of strength and a lack of wisdom. You cannot decide things in time because you lack determination, willpower, and one-pointedness. All success in the external and internal world depends on these factors. As you progress from one step to another it is very important to understand the mind and how it functions, for it functions in exactly the way you make it. The day you understand this and determine to change it, it changes of its own accord. So you must understand one more principle: determination.

Once you have analyzed and decided what to do, then you should determine to carry it out. Determination is the sixth principle. It should not be confused with obstinacy: determination expands, but obstinacy contracts. Determination is slowly and gradually built by the willpower of a one-pointed mind. Developing willpower is like letting an internal earning grow. Just as one earns money, puts it in savings, and is called rich when the interest mounts, so you should let your mind become rich from the willpower within you. Your willpower is at your disposal if your mind is one-pointed and concentrated. The more dissipation you have, the less willpower you have. And a dissipated mind is a constant source of stress.

Developing the skills of one-pointedness and determination is very simple, and you don't have to sit down and meditate to learn them: you can practice them while completing the activities of your everyday life. All you have to do is understand one thing: whenever you do anything, do it with full attention. No matter what you do, you should pay attention to it.

When you pay attention you will find that you have improved your concentration, or one-pointedness. No matter how many mantras you have, no matter how many gurus you claim, you will never learn meditation by just sitting in a corner for fifteen minutes and then remaining uncontrolled the rest of the day. Doing something halfheartedly means that you are distracted. You must learn to pay full attention to what you are doing all of the time. This is a sign of growth. Paying full attention will make you aware of the quality of your work. Then, later, you can analyze it: "I have done this much, but to raise the fruits of my actions properly, I should have done more." All mental powers such as psychic powers, mind control, voluntary control, getting a hunch, and going to the source of intuition depend upon one faculty: the faculty of determination. With this strength you can work with yourself to create physical, mental, and spiritual health.

When you learn to become a self-healer, to think positively, you can progress. When you start dealing with your mind and giving it an object to focus upon, this focusing of mind is called concentration. When you have developed the ability to focus the mind, then you learn to expand that ability: this is called meditation. Without expansion of your consciousness you do not grow; you remain within the boundaries which you have built with your petty desires and narrow-mindedness. Expansion is a law of life, and to go against it is to create more ignorance for yourself.

When you have analyzed the situation, decided what to do, and determined to do it, then you should take action. If you do that you will not fail—but if you do not take that final step even when you know what to do and how to do it, then you have not succeeded. Having true knowledge means that you know what to do, that you know how to do it—and that you do it at the right time. There is a Sanskrit word, *apta*, which means "a person who does and says whatever they think." Thinking, saying, and doing are the same for such a knowledgeable person. If you do not act, then you are not experimenting on what you have analyzed and decided in your thinking process. This means that you are not wholly confident. If you are not confident, you cannot be self-reliant, for self-reliance comes when you have performed action. Then, and only then, can you weigh your own capacity.

Through meditation you can control that part of the mind you use in daily life. When your consciousness starts moving upward you become aware of another level of life, and you understand more and more. If you do not meditate you do not know how to expand your consciousness; you have a narrow vision, as if you were looking through a window. But when you learn to expand your consciousness, it is like going through a door.

It is exactly as if you were looking through a small window in a house: from the window your view is very limited. But when you go out of the house you have a much wider view—and when you go to the roof you can see even more clearly. By the same token, as your consciousness expands, your vision becomes clearer, and you understand things as they are. In samadhi, you learn to expand your consciousness, fathom all boundaries, and unite yourself with the cosmic consciousness.

So through regular practice, patience, observation, analysis, discrimination, determination, and proper action, the mind becomes concentrated, and a concentrated mind can meditate very nicely. At last you reach the state of samadhi, the state of tranquility in which you do things yet remain above them. Nothing can affect you. Then, as your consciousness goes to the height of samadhi, your wisdom increases more and more, until complete transformation to a state of perfection takes place. This is the state of perfect stillness.

CHAPTER SIX

Emotions

*P*EOPLE FREQUENTLY TALK ABOUT knowing the mind and its various faculties, but they don't talk about feeling. Yet how can you know something without feeling it? When you perceive something, the first thing you are aware of is sensation. If you are not feeling something, you cannot know it. And if you lose the power to feel, you become insensitive. Those who are insensitive, who are not very emotional, who have learned to intellectualize everything, cannot become creative. They do not realize that beneath the thinking process lies the real source of creativity, which is emotion.

The right use of thinking is expression, but the right use of emotion is creativity. Emotion is a very great power: it is the highest power in your possession. When it comes to emotion, all human beings are one and the same—because intelligence has no place before it. When you become emotional you find that your reason has left you and that you cannot help yourself. When you are emotionally upset you become blind, you lose the power of discrimination, and your entire behavior—mind, action, and speech—becomes abnormal. Misuse of emotion is destructive, but this does not mean that all emotional power in itself is destructive. Those who are very emotional can become very creative if their emotions are properly guided and if they learn to direct them in a constructive way. People who know how to use their emotions creatively become successful in the external world and remain happy.

When emotion is led by devotion it is called ecstasy. The greatest things in the world have been done by people at the height of ecstasy. This is the work of emotion, not of the mind. Your intellectual gymnasium is not helpful in knowing your internal states. Though your mind is a very essential and powerful tool, it contains nothing new or original. It can only serve as far as the world of facts is concerned. Creativity and discovery lie beyond the mind. Emotion is the bridge between consciousness and creative thought. So you should learn to use the power of emotion to go beyond the limitations of thought.

Among the various functions of the mind, the intellect seems to be the finest—but without the help of emotional power the intellect is like a lame man who is not capable of reaching his destination. Even the highest of intellectuals can be suddenly disturbed by emotional outbursts. The untrained intellect has no power to check emotion. Those who have examined the external world ultimately find that there is something more to know and discover. They then turn within and start understanding their internal states. To do this they first need to make their mind one-pointed, and then become aware of the fact that the emotional level is deeper than the level of thoughts. When the mind is made one-pointed and inward it becomes lost, and finds itself incapable of fathoming the deeper and more subtle levels of inner life without the help of emotional power. So you cannot understand your entire personality by means of the thinking process alone, but you can do so by knowing the power of your emotions.

Though emotion is a great power, it needs to be directed willfully; otherwise it disturbs the mind. Our emotional body is like a fish in the lake of life. If the lake is in turmoil, it is impossible for the fish to remain calm and quiet. Similarly, if the mind is in constant turmoil, the emotions can never rest, and you can never use them correctly. The mind and emotions are very close, yet they are different in their functions. In the Sanskrit language the mind is called *manas* and emotion is called *bhava*. Let us discuss the origin of the emotions and see how we can make the best use of this power.

It is *kama*, the prime desire, that creates turmoil in the lake of life. *Kama* is the mother of all emotions. Since desire itself is mixed with selfishness, *kama* does not motivate you to serve others but instead controls your life and makes you self-centered. It builds a boundary around you and isolates you from the whole. The more you have that desire, *kama*, the more you contract your personality and are prevented from expanding your level of consciousness.

So desire is the prime factor of all motivations, and actions are performed according to the types of your desires. When you want to fulfill a desire you think, come to a conclusion, and then act accordingly. There are a variety of desires—active, passive, positive, negative—in the conscious and unconscious mind, and they come up to the surface and disturb the thinking process. But as it is important to understand the thinking process, it is even more important to understand the emotions which can disturb the thinking process. You can easily understand your inner being by finding out what types of desires you have.

All desires arise from four primitive fountains: self-preservation, sleep, food, and sex. As far as these fountains are concerned, human beings and animals are alike. A human being sleeps, takes food, has sex, and is always concerned with self-preservation; so also is the case with animals. The difference is that in the animal kingdom all activities are controlled and governed by nature, whereas human beings have the willpower to regulate and ultimately control these four appetites, and thus they are superior to all other living creatures in the world.

The strongest of the four primitive fountains is self-preservation. People are always trying to protect themselves; they are afraid because they don't want to die. In a calamity such as an earthquake I have even seen mothers leave very young children and run away to protect themselves because of their strong desire to live. The biggest fear is the fear of death; it is one thing that haunts us all the time: "What will happen to me if I die, if my wife dies?" Most people are insecure all the time because of this fear. But dying is a natural process, and all relationships are temporary because of it. This is true; and if the truth makes you insecure, then you are never safe anywhere you go. For nothing can make you secure if the truth cannot. But the truth is that there is no security anywhere. It is better for you to live with the truth than to live with insecurity. Insecurity that comes from the truth is good, and you will eventually enjoy it.

While all great people have achieved a state of fearlessness, most people live under the pressure of fear all the time. All fears are self-created; they come from a desire to obtain something which you are not fully equipped to attain. Fears develop in the mind, and if they are not examined and understood, they grow. If you keep all your fears within, then you will become neurotic. The main root of all dangers is fear, and the habit of being afraid actually invites danger. I once had an experience which illustrates this point:

I used to sit on a bank of the Ganges before dawn every day. When the sun rose I would stand, and then sit down again. One morning when I sat back down someone shouted, "Don't move! There is a snake beneath you!" The moment I heard that, I jumped and ran. Then the snake started chasing me! It chased me for fifty yards.

Later I went to one of the swamis and said, "This place is very dangerous. There are snakes that chase you." But he replied, "No. Your mind was chasing the snake, and you were actually mentally dragging it behind you. Your mind was negatively concentrated instead of positively concentrated."

Whenever you have a fear you are inviting danger by imagining it in your mind and then preparing for it. By doing this your mind becomes negatively one-pointed, and then that fear is not under your control. When you study the mind you will come to know the positive and negative aspects it contains. The negative mind has exactly as much power in being destructive as the positive mind has in being useful. That is why fears which are unexamined grow stronger and stronger every day until finally you lose your self-reliance.

You can learn to be fearless. But to develop fearlessness, internal strength is needed, because truth and fearlessness walk hand in hand. In order to achieve the state of fearlessness you must first examine the nature and cause of your fears. To examine your own fears closely you will have to go beyond your thinking process. When you do this you will find that the greatest fear is that of fear itself. But fear really doesn't exist at all! It is like darkness, which is actually only the absence of light. The sun has never seen darkness. It is they who do not see who are in the dark.

So you should learn to look at your fears and examine them properly.

Just as fear can cause discoordination between the mind, body, and senses, similar effects can be noticed from irregularities in sleep, the second primitive fountain. Sleep is a daily feature for everyone, rich or poor, and everyone continues to sleep throughout their whole life. But most of us do not know why we sleep, and few of us even analyze what it is. Sleep is a great pacifier, a state of rest which restores us every day. It is very important. If your sleep is disturbed you will get angry, your nervous system will remain very tense, and you will not work well. If you do not sleep properly you will be full of fears and will think that everyone is your enemy. If you don't get the rest which sleep provides you will remain in this same mood every day, and may even become insane. You will not be able to maintain your equilibrium.

It is very unhealthy to go to sleep when you are upset or have been talking crossly, because such sleep will not be refreshing. Instead you should walk, read, meditate, pray, or in some way resolve your differences and try to find solutions for your problems before you go to sleep. You should not go to sleep with many problems on your mind; the mind should be free from conflicting thoughts before you go to bed. Going to bed with many unresolved thoughts prompts you to have bad, nerve-shattering dreams. Restless sleep and dreams full of bad experiences are not healthy.

Of all the joys in the world, the most enjoyable is sleep. Two people make love and think that this is their finest joy—but then what do they do? They go to sleep. Sleep is the advanced state of joy. But people do not know how to sleep. In ordinary sleep any harsh sounds will make a bump in the sleep pattern and disturb the sleeper. However, there is one very good technique for sleeping, which will avoid this. It is called yogic sleep. This is sleep with full determination: no matter how many drums are beaten near a person who is in yoga sleep, they won't awaken. No one can wake them except themselves.

It is a myth that one should sleep for eight hours a day. The average person who works hard can curtail their sleep to three or four hours, and that will be sufficient. But those hours should be spent in deep sleep, not in dreaming, thinking, or waking. Sleeping for eight or ten hours is a bad habit. It wastes much time, and there is so much work to do, the finest being meditation. When a person has to plan for the next day, when they have to attain the state of tranquility, why should they waste time in disturbed sleep?

One of the finest principles of good health—which is very difficult for people nowadays—is waking up early in the morning. Pick up any book of poetry today: there is not a single poem on the rising sun. It's as if not a single poet has awakened in time to write about the rising sun within the last fifty years. After Shakespeare, Shelley, and Keats, who talks about the morning sun? Recent poets never talk about the dawn. Instead they talk about how beautiful the evening clouds are—sunset, evening dances, evening music—everything is evening and nothing is morning. But you should learn to get up early in the morning. Before the sun rises, you should rise from your bed.

There are certain times in the early morning when the ultraviolet rays of the sun have properties which help the skin. There are skin diseases which cannot be cured by medicine, but which can be cured by the sun's rays. So it is very important to wake up in the morning and do exercises before the sun. When you form the habit of sleeping too long you are filled with drowsiness, and that habit is called laziness or sloth. By making yourself lazy in this way, you create much unhappiness for yourself.

Food is the third primitive fountain of emotion. Poor food habits can make you emotionally upset and physically ill. The first control spiritual teachers will impress upon their students is control of the palate: you should look for the food value in what you eat, not the taste. In their instructions the teachers use a bitter pill with a blessed effect—but the world uses a sweet pill with a poisonous effect. Your food habits can make you emotionally upset, insecure, and sick—or, if you take food properly, you can avoid this. Being obsessed with food can have many causes. Sometimes those who do not eat the food which is essential for their body become emotionally disturbed and think of food all the time. One may also be compensating for a problem with one of the other primitive urges by overeating. Some people become "foodaholics"—they eat constantly. This is a danger, because food cannot be digested properly if the digestive system is never given a chance to rest. In taking food you should examine your capacity, act according to what is helpful in attaining your purpose in life, and maintain a state of cheerfulness.

Just as food should be regulated, so should sex, the fourth primitive urge. It should neither be overdone nor suppressed, since doing either can create many nervous and mental diseases. Sex is the least strong of the primitive urges; it is the only one we can live without. There is no doubt that sex is a very powerful urge, but it is not the most important. The reason it often appears to be so important is that it is more related to the mind than the other three urges. It is also most related to our relationships with other people. The sex act needs emotional control. People should prepare themselves mentally and unconsciously for having sex. A regular date and time should be set for this. By regulating your sex habits your mind does not run to the grooves of sexual thoughts all the time.

Sexual obsession and frustration are equally harmful. If you repress yourself sexually, or if your sexual life is not happy, this frustration will show itself in actions relating to one of the other primitive fountains, such as overeating. You should analyze your desires and regulate your habits according to your capacity and the purpose of life.

If these four primitive fountains are controlled they can be the source of good health and longevity, and eventually you will be able to regulate your thinking process and all of your emotions. If they are not regulated they will be the source of many problems and diseases.

You should learn to be peaceful while going to sleep, to be cheerful while taking food, and to be fully under control while engaging in sex. Otherwise, problems can be created in your mind. Anyone who wants to enjoy life can enjoy it in a better way if these appetites are regulated. If you have emotional problems you are making a mistake somewhere in controlling one of the urges, because all problems come from them. It is not difficult to know the source of problems if you learn to observe these four primitive fountains. Those who have regulated the four primitive urges have control over their emotions, and those who have emotional maturity are successful in the world and can be successful in enlightening themselves and attaining the purpose of life, which is self-perfection.

You should learn to observe your capacity and to be aware of one concept: no extremes. Those who are extremists do not know how to establish control over their appetites for food, sleep, and sex. If you know how to regulate these appetites you will surely lead a healthy life. Regulation helps the system and tunes it into the natural laws. Regulation does not mean abstention; it means balance based on examination of your capacity. Oversleeping or undersleeping, overindulging in sex or sexual repression, overeating or too much fasting—all are injurious to your health and your spiritual aspirations. They weaken the mind, create guilt feelings, and make you lose confidence.

When you study the emotions you find that there are seven main streams of negative emotions that arise from the four primitive fountains or appetites. Desire, or *kama*, which we have already discussed, is the first stream and the mother of them all.

Anger is the second stream. It is the expression of frustration for a desire that finds obstruction in its fulfillment. You should try to remember this whenever you get angry. Anger is different from what many modern therapists suggest. They say, "Come on, release your anger; let it out." It is true that if you do not express your anger it will turn into another disastrous direction; so you can let it out momentarily for the sake of your health. However, when you become angry your nervous system is activated, and in a fit of anger you might start acting like a wild animal. If you were to get angry all the time, you would want to express this anger all the time, and there would be no end to it; you would be forming a very bad habit. Anger is such a blind emotion that at its peak one can commit suicide or kill others. If you allowed yourself to release all your angers, you would be behind bars in a day. All the negative emotions are blind, but anger is the most dangerous.

Therefore it is very important to know how to train yourself not to get angry. This can definitely be done: it will happen when you learn how to control your desires. You should decide which desires are helpful for your growth and which desires will create obstructions to your growth. Learning to train the intellect within (*buddhi*) will definitely help in doing this: when you get angry, you can arrive at the source of your frustration and anger by sitting down and analyzing why you got angry in the first place and examining which desires were not fulfilled.

The third stream of negative emotion which is harmful for unfoldment arises when your desire is fulfilled and you become proud. "I have fulfilled my desires and others could not fulfill theirs. Look at how great I am." Pride happens when you have something others do not have and you are constantly aware of this.

The fourth emotion occurs when someone else succeeds in attaining the object of your desire, and you do not. This is called jealousy. You may have something—but someone else may have something you think is better. You find yourself incapable of fulfilling your own desires if the other person is fulfilling theirs. When you are jealous you are condemning yourself for being incompetent. You have lost the battle and accepted defeat.

The fifth emotion comes when you have something and you become attached to it by identifying yourself with it. You don't see its true nature: that it will go to decay, to destruction, to death; you become so attached that you don't realize this. For instance, a man has a wife, and as long as she is fulfilling all his desires he remains pleased with her. But the moment she loses her beauty, he gets upset. This is called attachment. Nowadays people do not seem to know the distinction between attachment and love. Attachment is selfish; love is selfless. Attachment brings bondage; love gives freedom. Attachment contracts consciousness; love expands it. Attachment becomes a source of torment; love becomes a source of liberation.

When two people meet, they should come together in grand liberation and joy, not in bondage and attachment. Misery comes because of attachment, because there is no giving in the relationship. The greatest happiness in life comes from giving, and the greatest chaos comes when two people claim to love each other but are really attached. Such a relationship, which is built on expectation, can only bring misery. When you really learn to love somebody you will be doing things selflessly and spontaneously, for love is that concern in which you enjoy giving and don't expect anything in return. That is the way to freedom.

The sixth emotion comes from attachment. It inspires you to want more and more. It is a perverted cultural desire which comes through competition and insecurity. It makes you narrow, selfish, self-centered, and petty-minded. It is called greed. Greedy people do not want to share the object of their attachment with others; they want to protect it.

The seventh emotion is the last and most powerful. It is egotism, which leads you to separate yourself from the whole by comparing yourself to others. Many times this is based on false pride: you are afraid because there may be somebody better than you. People who don't have anything frequently become egotistical to compensate for their inferiority complexes.

By examining these seven streams of emotion—desire, anger, pride, attachment, greed, jealousy, and egotism—you can analyze yourself. By studying your thoughts, speech, and actions you can find out how emotionally mature you are. All control is emotional. If the emotions are not controlled, there is no control at all. Control does not mean suppression of expression—it means regulation and balance within your capacity. With the help of reason and observation you can remain beyond the sway of emotion.

You should learn to attain a state of emotional maturity in which you know how to use your emotions positively. Positive emotion leads you to self-reliance and self-confidence, and motivates your mind, action, and speech in a joyous and creative way. Unselfish love is the highest positive emotion, and it can lead to devotion. When you love another, you want to serve and give to the loved one. You are prepared to give that person anything you possess. Such joy is a positive emotion, and helps you in being creative and in becoming a success in life. It results in peace, tranquility, and equilibrium.

Positive emotion is very helpful in self-growth. It has its roots in selfless service and love for others. This expands the human consciousness. When the mind tires of analyzing and searching for the answer to certain problems, positive emotion can help and lead the mind to a state of attainment. Those who are "insiders" and know the value of life, with its currents and crosscurrents, understand that the inner world has much to offer, and the more they dive deep into the inner levels the more they become aware of their human resources. When the four primitive urges are regulated and the seven streams of emotion are controlled, the positive emotions emerge. Then you can make the best use of your emotional power—which is the highest of all human powers—and can attain the highest wisdom. You should learn to attain a state of emotional maturity in which you know how to use your emotions positively.

By training yourself on the level of desire you can come to understand your inner nature. When you do this you will become aware of that which is called conscience. When you understand your conscience you will realize that it is like a mirror which can never lie. If you tell your conscience "I am a liar, but you must say that I am not a liar," your conscience will not be able to do it. If you paint your face, your mirror will always tell you which color it is painted. Even if the whole world tells you what a wonderful person you are, your conscience will know if you are a fake; no matter how much you implore it to lie, your conscience will still tell you the truth.

Modern man is trying to kill his conscience. We rely on feedback from others and are afraid of becoming aware of ourselves as we really are. This is because as we learn to understand ourselves from within we first come in touch with that part of our personality which we have been condemning, and then we identify ourselves with these negative thoughts. Such negative thinking is a constant source of disease. Condemning yourself and continually saying "I'm sorry" creates a sorry personality and a sorry state of health. Every time you feel bad and sorry you should learn to recognize and appreciate your own inner potential. Your internal and external conflicts weaken you until you have no capacity to enjoy the positive qualities within yourself.

You should never condemn yourself for thinking a particular thought. If you think of killing somebody you should remember that you are not actually killing anyone; you are only entertaining a thought, and you can let it pass away. You should not identify yourself with your thoughts. You are not a criminal for having bad thoughts. You become a criminal when you identify yourself with those thoughts and start acting according to them—but not before that. If you let the thoughts pass away, they are gone. So the thing for which you condemn yourself is really nothing. There is no way to overcome self-condemnation except to rely on your own inner mirror, your conscience. Going against your conscience is suicide.

Not a single emotion exists that is not related to something else. There is always some external object involved. Not a single emotion is your own. When you take in a sensation, the sensation finally leads to emotion. Emotion means relationship, and relationship means life. As long as you do not participate in life you will remain lonely. Loneliness is the root cause of many, many diseases. In a way, everyone is lonely. Though they are admiring and hugging each other, claiming how much they love and are loved, people are actually lonely. If you analyzed that loneliness you would find an amazing thing: you would find that it is those who love you who make you lonely. No stranger has the power to do that. Your loneliness means that your emotions are not under your control, that there is something wrong in your relationships. You should learn to be strong. Strength means not to be influenced by the suggestions and influence of others, especially by their negative suggestions. Positive suggestions become part of learning, but negative suggestions become part of self-destruction.

You can analyze any emotional problem you have—but analysis alone is not going to transform your personality if you don't train yourself. Following your conscience will help you to appreciate yourself and keep you from doing further damage. That is also a good beginning, but it will not undo the habits that are already formed. So you need to have a self-training program to change yourself. If you don't, you may know your problems but you will not be able to get rid of them. For instance, if you know that your pain lies at a specific spot, that knowledge is not going to help you much: you must learn the way to eliminate it. Everyone already has that ability within; you need only to become aware of the inner reality and come in touch with those potentials within you which will lead to a state of perennial happiness.

CHAPTER SEVEN

Self-Training

*A*LL HUMAN BEINGS want to attain a state of happiness that is free from all pains and fears. This can be attained by practicing a self-training method. The ancients described such a program in the traditional yogic manuscripts; it provides us with a way to reach a state of health on all levels. In following this program we learn through direct experience, and that alone is valid; it cannot be challenged by anyone. Most people are influenced by the opinions of others; they rarely take the opportunity to form their own opinions. Suggestion has been the very basis of modern life, and few of us draw our conclusions from direct experience. But without having direct experience, the information that we gather from external forces always remains questionable. That is why we need confirmation from others. Even in our relationships at home we expect others to tell us that it is good to do this or that: "You look good"; "Your clothes are nice"; "You speak well." These expressions show that we constantly seek the confirmation and appreciation of others because we are not sure on our own that we are doing well.

Once you have direct experience, however, you will be sure of your own actions. Direct experience does not need any evidence to prove its validity. When you have direct experience no external force can ever influence you, no matter how strong it is. The suggestions and opinions of others will not affect you then. For abstract knowing alone is not true knowledge: you obtain true knowledge only when you start experiencing. So in the program described by the ancient masters you are actually your own textbook, and you compare your own experience with that of the sages to verify the theories they give.

Self-training for self-knowledge works through experience, and although it is very subtle, it can bring you to the finest level of understanding possible. It is the best of all therapies. As human beings, we all need it because we do not know what situations may arise in the future, and we should be fully equipped to cope with them, whatever they may be. In a self-training program you train yourself. You are your own master and your own student: you play both roles. If the student is very conscientious and the teacher is very honest, then they can grow together.

For many years I have worked with people in therapy programs. They all start out by saying, "Let me see the doctor." But no health program in the world will ever be successful if the patient remains dependent upon the doctor, because then the patient will always be a patient and the doctor will always remain in the role of doctor. If you want to train yourself books, teachers, and other external aids are fine—but you have to learn for yourself, you have to involve yourself in a learning program. Getting training from a teacher, going to a seminar for a few days, and then saying, "It was good; I learned many things," is not completely helpful in itself, even if it was an inspiring program. You are still not fully educated. The real program for self-education begins when you start adding to these external sources yourself, getting into it, feeling, participating, realizing. Otherwise happiness, perfection, and samadhi are just words which you read in books: you know how to spell them, but you do not grasp their meaning. A human being has all the resources within needed to attain the highest state of wisdom.

If you do not study yourself through direct experience you will be dependent all the time on the opinions of others; you will never have a chance to experience the cause of things for yourself. For example, suppose you go to your teacher and say, "I had a psychic experience; what do you think about it?" The moment you ask the question or seek confirmation, it means that there is some doubt in your mind—but an experience which is conclusive in itself does not need any verification. It becomes the guide of your life. Then you can become fearless. You should go through self-examination, self-analysis, and self-training, for this is the simplest way to gain self-understanding and perfect health on all levels.

One of the greatest problems in human life is that we are often motivated to do things without fully understanding why we are doing them. People are always suggesting that we do things. For instance, if you are in pain and there is no doctor around, everybody will tell you about some medicine you should take or some special treatment you should have. You become caught up by their suggestions and don't use your common sense; you don't use your own mind to decide for yourself what you should do. You should not allow yourself to become dependent upon the opinions of others. You should do what you think, not what others think. Yet neither should you be so egotistical that you fail to hear and evaluate suggestions, since proper interaction with others is also very important.

You should accept the idea that you will train yourself, but you should not make any big resolutions. Small things are the best to start with. To begin with, you should improve yourself by learning to be kind and gentle right at home with the people you love. A husband should be a very good husband; a wife should be a very good wife. Just trying to do that is a sign of growth. You should let those you love see these signs of growth, and then watch your own development and enjoy it. Just as you watch a child grow, you should learn to see your improvement growing as a little spiritual child inside yourself.

Practicing spirituality should not cripple your daily duties. You should practice assimilation, gently adopting new habits to help your spiritual growth. If, for the sake of practice, you divide your life into two worlds, internal and external, then progress will become very easy. You will find yourself in a situation of gradual transformation, not of sudden change. You should not expect change; you should not expect that after working with yourself your appearance will change. That will not happen. But transformation is possible. Transformation is not change; it is growth. When you learn to transform your personality, then you will understand both your inner conditions and the world around you.

The first day you practice you will discover that your personality is made up of the thinking process, or outer life, and the emotions, or inner life. You should leave the inner personality aside at first and deal with the external behavior. In this way you can direct your mind, action, and speech. You should learn to speak less and not jabber uselessly. When you direct that energy which is now running along many avenues to the external world, you can do what you want. Sometimes merely a wish will make something happen, for that wish can be so powerful that the event will take place of itself. Nothing happens in the external world that has not already happened in the inner world. A plant will not sprout if the seed has not already begun to grow inside its shell. All things that are happening on the outside have happened within long before. But willing something and using willpower are two different things. For instance, if you will to do something, and then cannot do it, it is because there is no power supporting that will. There is no determination. If you have firm determination, with no distraction and no obstruction, then your willpower can create anything in the world.

When I was young I once asked my master, "What is free will?" He said, "Go and stand there." So I went and stood firmly on my two legs. Then he said, "Stand on one leg." So I did it. Then he said, "Now lift both legs." I said, "It is not possible!"

He said, "You have fifty percent of your will at your direct disposal. So first you should learn to use that. The other fifty percent will come to you when you have learned to use the first fifty percent." When you want to do something and cannot find the power to support the will, then it doesn't happen. When there is power behind it, then it happens. So learning to use your free will with determination and creativity is the next step in training yourself.

Whenever a problem comes up, you should not try to escape from it: you should learn to face it. When you face it, you will find that it is not so bad—but if you try to escape from it, it will create more and more problems for you. Wherever you go you will find new disturbances, but you cannot anticipate what those problems will be. You cannot escape from the disturbances of life, so running away will not help. Therefore your problems should be faced boldly and honestly.

Next, you should learn to be honest with yourself.

Being honest means learning to listen to yourself from within. In fact, the purpose of all the great scriptures of the world is to help you be aware of and in touch with that part within which is called the conscience. Their purpose is to introduce you to yourself, to that part of yourself which only you can know. Following your conscience strengthens your power of intuition. It is the first step toward spirituality.

After this, you should learn the philosophy of love or detachment. This will bring peace. This does not mean renunciation or depriving yourself of the things of the world, but it does mean not being absorbed by the world, not being lost in it. You should remain above. Then you can love anything that comes to you as a means to gain your goal. No matter what happens you should be constantly aware of your goal to maintain tranquility. You should learn to balance the world within and the world outside.

But you must understand more about your inner world, because you are a citizen of that true inner origin. If you relate to people properly, do your duties in the external world, know the art of living in the external world, and are still not happy within, then you are not balanced, for you are not tranquil and cannot be considered to be a whole person. Tranquility does not come from either isolating yourself from or losing yourself in the world. These two extremes are not healthy for human growth. Your attitude in the external world should be balanced—and in the internal world your awareness of the center of reality should be increased more and more and more. It is easy to act in the external world if you can remain aware of the reality within. So you should learn how to perform your actions while remaining aware of this inner reality all the time.

There are two principles which can help you do this.

The first is to become self-reliant. If you are not happy, you should not expect others to give you happiness. Happiness can never be given by anyone. This is the only concept which can help you be happy in the world, and if you don't grasp it—if you don't really learn it—then you will never be happy. If anybody claims that they can give someone else happiness, it is not true. Nobody can give happiness to anyone; they can, at best, only create patches of happiness for them. It is just as if something should happen to your own house. A neighbor might come and help you patch it. But if you were to depend too much on others, after some time you would be thanking everybody and those thanks would become a curse. You would realize that your whole house was nothing but patches and that it was no longer a sound structure. One day it would collapse. So you should do the rebuilding yourself and not depend on others; otherwise you will let yourself become a house of patches.

You should be self-reliant and learn how to make yourself happy. Many people expect others to make them happy—but they are never happy no matter how much others try to please them. Life is not limited to only the span that is seen. It is a long procession from the unknown to the unknown. Happiness is an attitude of mind coming out of an internal state of tranquility that allows you to go through that procession without disturbance. If you are expecting pleasure, you are also bound to have pain. Life is like a coin of which one side is pain and the other pleasure. You should realize these two inseparable opposites and accept life as it is. If you learn to be self-reliant, then you will be happy.

Practicing an internal dialogue is the second principle which can help you remain aware of the reality within while doing your actions in the world. You should sit down every morning and talk to yourself. This will help you learn more about yourself—and knowing about yourself, you will not become egotistical. All the ancient scriptures are dialogues. Christ talked with his apostles; Moses talked with the wise men; Krishna talked with Arjuna—these are all dialogues. You should also learn to go through a mental dialogue of your own. You could ask yourself, "Am I right? Am I really being fair?"

"Why do you feel bad? People say you are bad, but do you think you are? Do you want to accept this?"

"I think I have been bad, but it hurts me. I don't want to admit it."

"You are afraid of being hurt, and you don't want to realize that fact. This means you are weak."

"So how can I have strength?"

"Perhaps you should be honest. This dishonesty is draining your strength."

You should have this kind of dialogue with yourself within your mind every day. A conscious process of inner dialogue like this can pacify you and wash off all your bad feelings. This dialogue is one of the finest therapies there is, and prepares you for meditational therapy. Meditational therapy, if used and understood properly, is the highest of all the therapies, and teaches you how to be still on all levels: how to have physical stillness, a calm and even breath, and a calm, conscious mind. Then by allowing the unconscious mind to come forward you can go beyond it, and thus that inner reality comes to the conscious field and expands. You cannot explore the totality of the mind unless you apply the special technique called meditation—and unless you use that inward method you will never be able to understand yourself within. You will not be able to communicate, to relate to the external world, or to use your intelligence in a creative way. This ability comes through involving yourself in a self-training program.

When you begin to explore that inner world, you realize that the world within is larger than the world outside. Your outside world is actually very small—but when you close your eyes you can travel in your inner world to the sun, the moon, the stars. You can travel anywhere mentally, and you don't need anyone's help. You can create a great world within yourself, and it can have many levels. First of all you come in touch with the world of your own thoughts—but from where do those thoughts arise? It is like standing by the side of a lake and throwing a pebble into the water: that pebble will create many ripples, and after it has gone down to the bottom of the lake it will create bubbles; these bubbles will come up again and make more ripples. In the external world a sensation is just like a pebble in the lake of the mind: it leaves an impression within your mind and creates many bubbles; when it leaves a permanent impression, we call it memory.

When you are pursuing meditational therapy you first come in touch with those memories which are fresh; then you come in touch with those memories which are old; and then you come in touch with those formless memories which are sleeping within, which you have not been aware of until this time. Facts without forms cannot be remembered unless you come in touch with that part of the mind which is called the hidden mind. When you come in touch with that, it leads the way. When you experience this, it is like the fog rolling back from the world and into the ocean. An unborn chicken which remains inside the shell can never imagine what is outside—but when the shell is broken, the whole situation changes. You should learn to break that shell that you have created around yourself, for creating boundaries contracts the personality.

How do you realize that fact, that reality, which is beyond names and forms? When your mind is prepared for it, then you will start treading the path of spirituality and start enlightening yourself. This comes through your direct experience from within. It is not a creation; it is not an attainment.

How do we know what enlightenment is? We know because the great people who were born just like us, whose mothers were just like our mother, who walked on the earth, who were human beings, but who had enlightenment, told us what it is and how to reach it. Human beings do not understand that they are complete. They doubt their own existence—yet they want to believe in the existence of something which they have not realized, felt, or seen. They should learn to believe, appreciate, and admire their own existence first. That is what proves the reality of the existence of the Lord.

We are each a part of eternity. If God is omnipresent, then He is within us too. The day we come to know that all these boundaries are created by self-ignorance, absent-mindedness, and selfishness is the day we can break them and just be enlightened.

My master used to say, "You are already God, so don't try to know God. That godly part is already there in you. All you have to do is become fully human. That is your part to play—to be a good human being so that the reality called God can flow spontaneously." Human beings act abnormally and try to get enlightenment without understanding what it is. The greatest misery is that each of us has a home but has forgotten the way to get there. We do not identify ourselves with the reality of God within; we identify ourselves with that which seems to be convenient, which seems to comfort momentarily. But after going through many experiences in life we come to know that though we have a body, we are something far beyond it.

Enlightenment is an expansion of consciousness. When you become enlightened you become aware of something more than yourself, of something more than your own interest. The more you become aware of others the closer you come to the center, where you find that all diversities have an underlying unity. The diversities are only superficial layers of the one unity. There are many ornaments, but there is only one great goal. There are many waves, but there is only one water. All human beings are different, but they all inhale and exhale the same life-force. No matter what religion you come from, there is only one proprietor of all the different beings. When you consider this reality for some time, you start thinking, start understanding, start becoming aware of the truth.

If you want God to reveal Himself, He will—but first you have to create the proper conditions. If you were to go to a powerhouse with a lightbulb in your hand and ask, "Will you please light my bulb?" they could not do it. The power outlet is in your own house; this is where you have the switch and all the fittings. So why do you need power from outside when it is already there inside you? The powerhouse is within you. It is ready to give you power— but only when you have all the proper fittings. You are shouting, "O powerhouse, O powerhouse, please come to me!" But it is already there! All you need are a few of the fittings.

When you have truly understood yourself, you are one with the source of peace, bliss, and perennial happiness within. You have reached that state which is called enlightenment. And when you have done this, you become an instrument which can be played by the source within.

When you play the guitar you have to tune it first, and that is a painful thing for the guitar. If you really want to be enlightened, be prepared for this. All the parts of your body will have to be properly twisted and tuned because He wants to play. You cannot be selfish; if you are selfish and resist, you will break. You are exactly like a guitar which is being played. If you just let yourself become a willing instrument, there will be no problem.

About the Author

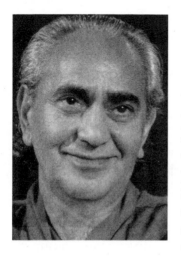

BORN IN 1925 in northern India, Swami Rama was raised from early childhood by a great Bengali yogi and saint who lived in the foothills of the Himalayas. In his youth he practiced the various disciplines of yoga science and philosophy in the traditional monasteries of the Himalayas and studied with many spiritual adepts, including Mahatma Gandhi, Sri Aurobindo, and Rabindranath Tagore. He also traveled to Tibet to study with his grandmaster.

He received his higher education at Prayaga, Varanasi, and Oxford University, England. At the age of twenty-four he became Shankaracharya of Karvirpitham in South India, the highest spiritual position in India. During this term he had a tremendous impact on the spiritual customs of that time: he dispensed with useless formalities and rituals, made it possible for all segments of society to worship in the temples, and encouraged the instruction of women in meditation. He renounced the dignity and prestige of this high office in 1952 to return to the Himalayas to intensify his yogic practices.

After completing an intense meditative practice in the cave monasteries, he emerged with the determination to serve humanity, particularly to bring the teachings of the East to the West. With the encouragement of his master, Swami Rama began his task by studying Western philosophy and psychology. He worked as a medical consultant in London and assisted in parapsychological research in Moscow. He then returned to India, where he established an ashram in Rishikesh. He completed his degree in homeopathy at the medical college in Darbhanga in 1960. He came to the United States in 1969, bringing his knowledge and wisdom to the West. His teachings combine Eastern spirituality with modern Western therapies.

Swami Rama was a freethinker, guided by his direct experience and inner wisdom, and he encouraged his students to be guided in the same way. He often told them, "I am a messenger, delivering the wisdom of the Himalayan sages of my tradition. My job is to introduce you to the teacher within."

Swami Rama came to America upon the invitation of Dr. Elmer Green of the Menninger Foundation of Topeka, Kansas, as a consultant in a research project investigating the voluntary control of involuntary states. He participated in experiments that helped to revolutionize scientific thinking about the relationship between body and mind, amazing scientists by his demonstrating, under laboratory conditions, precise conscious control of autonomic physical responses and mental functioning, feats previously thought to be impossible.

Swami Rama founded the Himalayan International Institute of Yoga Science and Philosophy, the Himalayan Institute Hospital Trust in India, and many centers throughout the world. He is the author of numerous books on health, meditation, and the yogic scriptures. Swami Rama left his body in November 1996.

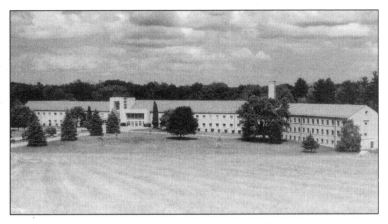

The main building of the Institute headquarters, near Honesdale, Pennsylvania.

The Himalayan Institute

FOUNDED IN 1971 by Swami Rama, the Himalayan Institute has been dedicated to helping people grow physically, mentally, and spiritually by combining the best knowledge of both the East and the West.

Our international headquarters is located on a beautiful 400-acre campus in the rolling hills of the Pocono Mountains of northeastern Pennsylvania. The atmosphere here is one to foster growth, increased inner awareness, and calm. Our grounds provide a wonderfully peaceful and healthy setting for our seminars and extended programs. Students from around the world join us here to attend programs in such diverse areas as hatha yoga, meditation, stress reduction, Ayurveda, nutrition, Eastern philosophy, psychology, and other subjects. Whether the programs are for weekend meditation retreats, week-long seminars on spirituality, months-long residential programs, or holistic health services, the attempt here is to provide an environment of gentle inner progress. We invite you to join with us in the ongoing process of personal growth and development.

The Institute is a nonprofit organization. Your membership in the Institute helps to support its programs. Please call or write for information on becoming a member.

Institute Programs, Services, and Facilities

Institute programs share an emphasis on conscious holistic living and personal self-development, including:

Special weekend or extended seminars to teach skills and techniques for increasing your ability to be healthy and enjoy life

Meditation retreats and advanced meditation and philosophical instruction

Vegetarian cooking and nutritional training

Hatha yoga and exercise workshops

Residential programs for self-development

Holistic health services and Ayurvedic Rejuvenation Programs through the Institute's Center for Health and Healing.

A *Quarterly Guide to Programs and Other Offerings* is free within the USA. To request a copy, or for further information, call 800-822-4547 or 570-253-5551, fax 570-253-9078, email bqinfo@himalayaninstitute.org, write the Himalayan Institute, RR 1 Box 400, Honesdale, PA 18431-9706 USA, or visit our Web site at www. himalayaninstitute.org.

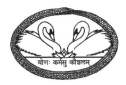

The Himalayan Institute Press

THE HIMALAYAN INSTITUTE PRESS has long been regarded as "The Resource for Holistic Living." We publish dozens of titles, as well as audio and video tapes, that offer practical methods for living harmoniously and achieving inner balance. Our approach addresses the whole person—body, mind, and spirit—integrating the latest scientific knowledge with ancient healing and self-development techniques.

As such, we offer a wide array of titles on physical and psychological health and well-being, spiritual growth through meditation and other yogic practices, as well as translations of yogic scriptures.

Our sidelines include the Japa Kit for meditation practice, the Neti™ Pot, the ideal tool for sinus and allergy sufferers, and The Breath Pillow,™ a unique tool for learning health-supportive diaphragmatic breathing.

Subscriptions are available to a bimonthly magazine, *Yoga International*, which offers thought-provoking articles on all aspects of meditation and yoga, including yoga's sister science, Ayurveda.

For a free catalog call 800-822-4547 or 570-253-5551, email hibooks@himalayaninstitute.org, fax 570-253-6360, write the Himalayan Institute Press, RR 1, Box 405, Honesdale, PA 18431-9709, USA, or visit our Web site at www.himalayaninstitute.org.